KATE HALE

Early Childhood Cognitive Development

Key Factors Shaping a Child's Thinking Abilities

Contents

INTRODUCTION

Cognitive development during early childhood is one of the most critical areas of growth, setting the stage for lifelong learning and adaptability. Understanding this process is essential for parents, caregivers, and educators, as it shapes the way children think, learn, and interact with the world around them. This book explores the various factors that influence a child's cognitive development and provides actionable insights that can be used to support optimal brain growth during these formative years.

Cognitive development encompasses more than just the acquisition of knowledge. It includes the development of reasoning, problem-solving, memory, attention, and language skills—abilities that allow a child to make sense of their experiences and surroundings. As a parent or caregiver, understanding these processes can empower you to create an environment that fosters healthy cognitive growth. With the right guidance and support, children can develop strong thinking abilities that will serve them well throughout their lives.

This book is structured to help readers navigate the complexities of early childhood cognitive development, breaking down key concepts into easily digestible sections. Each chapter addresses a specific factor that contributes to cognitive growth, from the role of nutrition and parental engagement to the impact of play and social interactions. The aim is to provide both a theoretical understanding of cognitive development and practical tools that can be implemented at home or in educational settings.

Through this exploration, we also address the challenges that may arise during a child's cognitive development. Developmental delays, learning disabilities, and the effects of socioeconomic factors are discussed, with a focus on how early intervention can help mitigate these issues. We also provide strategies for parents and educators to overcome these challenges, ensuring that every child has the opportunity to reach their full cognitive potential.

Cognitive development during the early years is not only a matter of individual growth but also a societal investment. By nurturing the intellectual capacities of young children, we lay the foundation for a more innovative, resilient, and emotionally intelligent future generation. In short, the cognitive development of children is vital not only for their personal success but also for the collective well-being of society.

Why Cognitive Development Matters

Cognitive development plays a pivotal role in shaping how children perceive, think, and interact with the world around them. It is through cognitive processes that children learn to understand cause and effect, recognize patterns, solve problems, and develop critical thinking skills. The importance of cognitive development cannot be overstated, as it forms the basis for academic success, social competence, and emotional regulation.

One of the key reasons why cognitive development matters is that it influences a child's ability to learn. Children who have strong cognitive abilities tend to excel in school, as they are better equipped to grasp new concepts, retain information, and apply knowledge in various contexts. On the other hand, children who experience cognitive delays may struggle with learning, leading to frustration, low self-esteem, and even behavioral issues.

In addition to academic success, cognitive development also impacts a child's social and emotional well-being. Children with well-developed cognitive skills are better able to regulate their emotions, understand social cues, and build positive relationships with others. They can empathize with others, navigate social challenges, and communicate their thoughts and feelings effectively. This emotional intelligence, which is closely tied to cognitive development, is crucial for forming healthy relationships and functioning successfully in a community.

Moreover, cognitive development is not limited to early childhood. It is a lifelong process, but the foundation laid during the early years is critical for future growth. The brain's plasticity, or its ability to change and adapt, is greatest during early childhood, making this period a unique window of opportunity for cognitive development. By providing children with the right experiences and stimuli, we can shape their cognitive abilities in ways that will benefit them throughout their lives.

The Critical Role of Early Years (Birth to Age 5)

The period from birth to age five is often referred to as the "critical period" for cognitive development. During these years, the brain undergoes rapid growth and development, forming the neural connections that will support future learning and thinking abilities. In fact, by the time a child reaches age five, their brain has reached 90% of its adult size, making early childhood a crucial time for cognitive development.

Several factors contribute to the brain's rapid development during the early years. Genetics play a role in determining a child's cognitive potential, but environmental factors are equally important. The experiences a child has during their early years—whether positive or negative—can have a profound impact on their brain development. Positive experiences, such as engaging in play, interacting with caregivers, and exploring new environments, can enhance cognitive development. On the other hand, negative experiences, such as neglect, abuse, or lack of stimulation, can hinder cognitive growth.

One of the most important aspects of cognitive development during the early years is the formation of synapses, the connections between neurons in the brain. These synapses are the pathways through which information is transmitted, and their formation is influenced by a child's experiences. The more a child is exposed to new stimuli, the more synapses their brain forms, allowing for greater cognitive flexibility and learning potential.

During this critical period, children also begin to develop the cognitive skills that will serve as the foundation for future learning. These skills include memory, attention, problem-solving, and language. Memory is essential for retaining information and applying it in new situations, while attention allows children to focus on tasks and filter out distractions. Problem-solving skills enable children to think critically and come up with solutions to challenges, and language development allows them to communicate their thoughts and ideas effectively.

The early years also set the stage for the development of executive function, a set of cognitive skills that includes self-control, working memory, and flexible thinking. These skills are essential for academic success, social interactions, and emotional regulation. For example, a child with strong executive function is better able to control their impulses, follow instructions, and adapt to changing situations. These skills are not fully developed during early childhood, but the foundation is laid during this critical period.

Goals of the Book: Supporting Parents, Caregivers, and Educators

This book is designed to be a comprehensive resource for parents, caregivers, and educators who want to support the cognitive development of young children. The goals of the book are threefold: to provide a clear understanding of the cognitive development process, to offer practical strategies for fostering cognitive growth, and to address the challenges that may arise during a child's development.

One of the main goals of the book is to demystify cognitive development and explain the science behind how children learn and think. Many parents and caregivers may feel overwhelmed by the complexity of brain development, but this book breaks down the key concepts in a way that is easy to understand. By gaining a deeper understanding of cognitive development, readers will be better equipped to create environments that support learning and intellectual growth.

In addition to providing a theoretical understanding of cognitive development, the book also offers practical strategies that can be implemented in everyday life. These strategies are based on the latest research in child development and are designed to be simple, actionable, and effective. Whether it's engaging in play, providing a nutritious diet, or creating a stimulating learning environment, the book provides readers with concrete steps they can take to support their child's cognitive development.

The book also addresses the challenges that parents, caregivers, and educators may face when it comes to cognitive development. Developmental delays, learning disabilities, and the effects of socioeconomic factors are all discussed in detail, with a focus on how early intervention can help mitigate these challenges. By providing readers with the tools and resources they need to overcome these obstacles, the book aims to ensure that every child has the opportunity to reach their full cognitive potential.

Finally, the book serves as a guide for educators who are working with young children in formal settings, such as preschools and daycare centers. The strategies outlined in the book can be easily adapted for use in the classroom, providing educators with the tools they need to create a rich and stimulating learning environment. By fostering cognitive development in the early years, educators can set the stage for future academic success and lifelong learning.

A Glimpse Into Cognitive Milestones

Cognitive development is a gradual process, and children reach different milestones at different ages. These milestones serve as markers of a child's cognitive growth and provide parents, caregivers, and educators with a general sense of what to expect at each stage of development.

During the first year of life, cognitive development is primarily focused on sensory and motor experiences. Infants begin to explore their environment through touch, sight, sound, and movement. They develop object permanence, the understanding that objects continue to exist even when they are out of sight, and they start to recognize patterns and make associations between actions and outcomes.

By the age of two, toddlers begin to develop more complex cognitive skills, such as symbolic thinking and language. They start to use words to represent objects and actions, and they engage in pretend play, which allows them to explore different roles and scenarios. Toddlers also begin to develop problem-solving skills, such as figuring out how to stack blocks or complete simple puzzles.

Between the ages of three and five, children continue to develop their cognitive abilities, with a focus on language, memory, and attention. They start to ask questions about the world around them, demonstrating a growing curiosity and desire to learn. Their memory improves, allowing them to recall information and events from the past, and their attention span increases, enabling them to focus on tasks for longer periods of time.

During this stage, children also begin to develop executive function skills, such as self-control and flexible thinking. They learn to follow rules, take turns, and manage their emotions in social situations. These skills are essential for success in school and in life, as they enable children to navigate challenges, work collaboratively with others, and adapt to new situations.

Cognitive development does not stop at age five, but the foundation laid during these early years is critical for future growth. By understanding the milestones of cognitive development and providing children with the support and stimulation they need, parents, caregivers, and educators can help children reach their full intellectual potential.

In conclusion, this book serves as a comprehensive guide to understanding and supporting cognitive development in early childhood. By exploring the factors that influence cognitive development and offering practical strategies for parents, caregivers, and educators, it aims to empower those involved in a child's early years to make informed decisions that positively impact a child's future. The insights provided throughout the book are designed to be both accessible and actionable, ensuring that readers can immediately apply the knowledge to everyday interactions with children.

By recognizing the importance of cognitive development and addressing the critical role of early experiences, this book underscores the idea that the foundation for lifelong learning is laid during the first five years of life. The brain's remarkable plasticity during these years means that the experiences and environments children are exposed to have a profound effect on how they think, learn, and grow. As such, it is crucial to provide children with rich, stimulating environments and supportive interactions that encourage cognitive growth.

The ultimate goal of this book is not only to inform but to inspire action. Parents, caregivers, and educators are on the front lines of shaping the cognitive trajectories of young children, and this book provides them with the tools and knowledge needed to make a significant difference. Whether it is through engaging in meaningful conversations, offering new learning experiences, or simply being present and supportive, the actions taken during a child's early years have lasting impacts.

As readers progress through the chapters, they will gain a deeper understanding of how each element—be it language, nutrition, play, or social interactions—contributes to a child's cognitive development. The book emphasizes that no one factor works in isolation; rather, it is the interplay of various influences that shape a child's thinking abilities. By fostering a holistic approach to cognitive development, readers will be better equipped to support the growth of well-rounded, curious, and resilient thinkers.

Ultimately, this book advocates for a proactive and intentional approach to raising and educating children. Cognitive development is a dynamic process, and by staying informed and involved, parents, caregivers, and educators can play a pivotal role in ensuring that children not only reach important developmental milestones but also thrive as lifelong learners. Through knowledge, understanding, and thoughtful action, we can all contribute to building the cognitive foundations that children need to succeed in an ever-changing world.

—-

The next chapters will delve into the specifics of how various factors influence cognitive development and provide detailed, evidence-based strategies that readers can use to nurture a child's growing mind. From language acquisition to problem-solving skills, each section is crafted to help readers understand the science behind cognitive development while providing practical insights they can apply immediately. By integrating the latest research with real-world applications, this book serves as a valuable resource for anyone invested in the cognitive development of young children.

What is Cognitive Development

Cognitive development refers to the process by which children acquire the ability to think, reason, understand, and learn. It is a fundamental aspect of childhood that shapes not only intellectual growth but also emotional and social development. In simple terms, cognitive development is the evolution of the brain's capacity to process information, make sense of the world, and respond to stimuli. This process begins at birth and continues throughout life, but the most rapid and significant changes occur during early childhood.

One of the most influential ways to understand cognitive development is through the study of developmental theories, which offer frameworks for understanding how children think and learn. These theories help us comprehend the stages and mechanisms through which cognitive growth occurs. Two of the most prominent theories in the study of cognitive development are those proposed by Jean Piaget and Lev Vygotsky.

Jean Piaget's theory of cognitive development suggests that children move through four distinct stages of mental development: the sensorimotor stage, preoperational stage, concrete operational stage, and formal operational stage. Each stage represents a different way of thinking and understanding the world. According to Piaget, children are not passive recipients of information; rather, they actively construct knowledge by interacting with their environment. This idea, known as constructionist, posits that learning is a process of building on prior knowledge through experience.

Piaget's sensorimotor stage, which occurs from birth to about two years, is characterized by infants learning through sensory experiences and manipulating objects. During this stage, children begin to understand object permanence—the realization that objects continue to exist even when they are not visible. The preoperational stage, which spans from ages two to seven, marks the development of symbolic thought, allowing children to use words and images to represent objects. However, Piaget noted that children in this stage are still limited by egocentrism, meaning they struggle to see things from perspectives other than their own.

The concrete operational stage, from ages seven to eleven, sees children develop logical thinking about concrete objects and events. They become capable of understanding concepts like conservation—the understanding that quantity remains the same even if its appearance changes. Finally, the formal operational stage, which begins at around age eleven and continues into adulthood, involves the ability to think abstractly, reason hypothetically, and engage in systematic problem-solving.

While Piaget's theory has been incredibly influential, it is not without its critics. Some researchers argue that his model underestimates the cognitive abilities of young children, suggesting that they may be capable of more advanced thinking at earlier ages than Piaget proposed. Nonetheless, his work remains a foundational aspect of understanding cognitive development.

Lev Vygotsky, another major figure in developmental psychology, offered a different perspective on cognitive development. His theory emphasizes the social context of learning and suggests that cognitive development is heavily influenced by interactions with others. Vygotsky introduced the concept of the "zone of proximal development" (ZPD), which refers to the range of tasks that a child can perform with the help of a more knowledgeable individual, such as a parent, teacher, or peer. According to Vygotsky, learning occurs in this zone when a child is supported by others to accomplish tasks that are just beyond their current abilities.

In contrast to Piaget's focus on individual exploration and discovery, Vygotsky believed that social interaction plays a crucial role in cognitive development. Through communication and collaboration with others, children learn cultural tools—such as language, symbols, and problem-solving strategies—that shape their thinking. Vygotsky also emphasized the importance of language in cognitive development, arguing that language is both a tool for communication and a mechanism for thought. This theory highlights the role of teachers, parents, and peers in guiding a child's learning and cognitive growth.

Both Piaget and Vygotsky's theories provide valuable insights into how children learn and think. While Piaget focuses on the child's individual exploration of their environment, Vygotsky emphasizes the importance of social interactions and cultural influences on learning. Together, these theories offer a more complete understanding of cognitive development, acknowledging both the internal and external factors that contribute to intellectual growth.

Children learn and think in complex ways that involve multiple processes working together. Cognitive development is not limited to a single domain, such as memory or language, but rather encompasses a range of skills that enable children to acquire, retain, and apply knowledge. Some of the key processes involved in cognitive development include attention, memory, language acquisition, problem-solving, and executive function.

Attention is a critical cognitive skill that allows children to focus on specific stimuli while ignoring distractions. The ability to sustain attention improves over time, enabling children to engage more deeply with tasks and learning experiences. Memory, another essential cognitive process, involves encoding, storing, and retrieving information. Young children develop memory skills rapidly, and their capacity to recall and use information grows as they age.

Language acquisition is a key aspect of cognitive development, as language provides the means for communication, thought, and learning. From babbling and cooing as infants to forming complete sentences as toddlers, children's language skills develop in tandem with their cognitive abilities. The acquisition of language also plays a significant role in shaping other cognitive processes, such as reasoning and problem-solving.

Problem-solving is a complex cognitive skill that involves identifying challenges and finding solutions. From a young age, children demonstrate problem-solving abilities by experimenting with different actions to achieve desired outcomes. For example, an infant may learn how to stack blocks by trial and error, while a preschooler may figure out how to complete a puzzle by applying patterns and strategies.

Executive function, a set of cognitive skills that includes self-control, working memory, and flexible thinking, is essential for managing thoughts, actions, and emotions. These skills enable children to plan, focus attention, remember instructions, and juggle multiple tasks. Executive function develops gradually and is influenced by both biological and environmental factors.

One of the most enduring debates in cognitive development is the role of nature versus nurture. Nature refers to the genetic and biological factors that influence cognitive development, while nurture encompasses the environmental factors, such as experiences, relationships, and culture, that shape a child's learning and thinking.

Research shows that both nature and nurture play significant roles in cognitive development. For example, a child's genetic makeup can influence their cognitive abilities, such as memory capacity or attention span. However, environmental factors, such as the quality of parental interactions, access to educational resources, and exposure to stimulating experiences, also have a profound impact on cognitive development.

The nature versus nurture debate has evolved over time, with most experts now agreeing that cognitive development is the result of a dynamic interplay between both genetic and environmental factors. Genes provide the foundation for cognitive development, but experiences and interactions with the environment shape how these genetic potentials are expressed. For example, a child may be born with the genetic predisposition for strong language skills, but the extent to which these skills develop will depend on the richness of their language environment—whether they are exposed to conversations, reading, and storytelling.

Cognitive milestones are key indicators of a child's cognitive development and provide a framework for understanding how thinking abilities evolve over time. While every child is unique and may reach milestones at different rates, these markers offer general guidelines for what to expect at various stages of early childhood.

From birth to age two, children experience rapid cognitive growth as they explore their surroundings and develop sensory and motor skills. During this period, children learn to interact with the world through their senses—touch, sight, hearing, taste, and smell. Object permanence, the understanding that objects continue to exist even when they are not visible, is a significant cognitive milestone that typically develops around eight to twelve months of age. By the end of this stage, children begin to engage in goal-directed behavior, such as reaching for a toy or crawling toward an object of interest.

Between the ages of two and four, children enter the preoperational stage of cognitive development, as described by Piaget. During this stage, children's thinking becomes more symbolic, and they begin to use language to represent objects and actions. They also engage in pretend play, which allows them to experiment with different roles and scenarios. However, their thinking is still limited by egocentrism, meaning they have difficulty seeing things from perspectives other than their own. Children in this age group also begin to develop the ability to classify objects based on shared characteristics, such as size, color, or shape.

From ages four to six, children's cognitive abilities continue to grow, and they begin to develop more logical thinking. They become better at understanding cause-and-effect relationships and can solve simple problems by applying basic reasoning skills. At this stage, children also start to understand concepts such as time, quantity, and numbers, although their understanding is still concrete rather than abstract. Their memory and attention span improve, allowing them to engage in more complex tasks and activities for longer periods.

It is important to note that while cognitive milestones provide a general framework for understanding development, every child is unique, and there is considerable variability in the rate at which children reach these milestones. Some children may reach certain cognitive milestones earlier or later than others, and this variation is often within the normal range of development. However, if a child shows significant delays in reaching cognitive milestones, it may be a sign of a developmental disorder or learning disability, and early intervention may be necessary to support the child's growth.

In conclusion, cognitive development is a complex and multifaceted process that involves the acquisition of skills such as attention, memory, language, problem-solving, and executive function. Theories by researchers such as Piaget and Vygotsky provide valuable insights into how children learn and think, highlighting the importance of both individual exploration and social interactions in shaping cognitive growth. The debate between nature and nurture underscores the idea that cognitive development is influenced by a combination of genetic and environmental factors, with experiences playing a crucial role in how children's thinking abilities unfold. By understanding the key processes and milestones of cognitive development, parents, caregivers, and educators can create environments that support and nurture a child's intellectual growth.

The Developing Brain

The human brain is an extraordinary organ, and its development in early childhood is one of the most complex and rapid processes in the human body. Understanding how the brain grows and forms connections is essential for anyone invested in fostering optimal cognitive development in young children. The brain's development begins long before birth and continues into adulthood, but the most significant changes occur in the early years, shaping how children think, learn, and interact with the world. As the brain grows, it not only increases in size but also in complexity, forming billions of connections that enable children to process information, solve problems, and make sense of their experiences.

During the early stages of development, the brain's growth is both quantitative and qualitative. Quantitatively, the brain increases in size, reaching approximately 80% of its adult volume by age two and around 90% by age five. However, the qualitative changes are even more remarkable. The brain consists of approximately 86 billion neurons, or brain cells, at birth. These neurons form synapses, or connections, with each other, creating the intricate neural networks that support cognitive functions. By age three, a child's brain has formed over a trillion synapses, far more than it will need as an adult. This overproduction of synapses allows for incredible flexibility in the developing brain, but many of these connections will eventually be pruned, or eliminated, based on a child's experiences.

The process of synaptogenesis, or the formation of synapses, is one of the key mechanisms by which the brain grows during early childhood. Synaptogenesis occurs rapidly in the first few years of life, with different areas of the brain developing at different rates. For example, the sensorimotor areas of the brain, which are responsible for processing sensory information and coordinating movement, develop earlier than the areas responsible for higher-order thinking, such as the prefrontal cortex. This difference in developmental timing reflects the brain's prioritization of essential functions—such as seeing, hearing, and moving—before more complex cognitive processes like decision-making and reasoning.

The formation of synapses is heavily influenced by a child's experiences. Every time a child has a new experience—whether it's touching a soft toy, hearing a parent's voice, or looking at a brightly colored object—the brain forms new connections to process that information. This experience-dependent synaptogenesis highlights the importance of providing children with a rich and stimulating environment during their early years. The more varied and engaging a child's experiences, the more connections their brain will form, leading to enhanced cognitive development.

While the brain is highly flexible and capable of forming new connections, it also undergoes a process of synaptic pruning, where unused connections are eliminated. This process is essential for brain efficiency, as it allows the brain to focus on strengthening the most important and frequently used connections. Synaptic pruning begins in early childhood and continues into adolescence, shaping the brain's structure based on a child's experiences. For example, if a child is frequently exposed to language, the neural pathways related to language processing will be strengthened, while unused pathways may be pruned. This process underscores the importance of early stimulation, as the connections that are reinforced during childhood will have lasting effects on cognitive abilities.

Critical periods in brain development refer to specific windows of time during which the brain is particularly sensitive to certain types of input or experiences. During these periods, the brain is highly plastic, meaning it can easily adapt and reorganize itself in response to stimuli. While the brain remains plastic throughout life, critical periods represent times of heightened sensitivity, during which the brain is especially receptive to learning and development in specific domains, such as language, vision, and motor skills.

One of the most well-known examples of a critical period is in language development. Research shows that children are most adept at acquiring language during the first few years of life. During this time, the brain is primed to learn the sounds, grammar, and structure of language. If a child is not exposed to language during this critical period, they may have difficulty fully acquiring language later in life, even with intervention. This phenomenon has been observed in cases of children who were deprived of language exposure due to neglect or isolation; these children often struggle with language acquisition even after being placed in a stimulating environment.

Similarly, vision is another area with a well-defined critical period. In early infancy, the brain is highly sensitive to visual input. If a child is deprived of visual stimulation, such as in the case of congenital cataracts, the brain's ability to process visual information may be permanently impaired, even if the cataracts are removed later. This underscores the importance of early detection and intervention in cases where visual development may be at risk.

Motor skills also develop during critical periods. Babies are born with reflexes that allow them to perform basic movements, such as sucking and grasping, but the refinement of motor skills—such as crawling, walking, and hand-eye coordination—occurs through practice and experience. The brain is particularly plastic during early childhood, making it an ideal time for developing gross and fine motor skills. If a child does not have opportunities to practice these skills during this critical period, they may face challenges in motor development later in life.

While critical periods represent windows of heightened sensitivity, it is important to note that the brain remains capable of learning and adapting throughout life. However, learning certain skills may become more difficult after the critical period has passed, as the brain becomes less plastic with age. This concept highlights the importance of providing children with enriching experiences during the critical periods of brain development, as it sets the foundation for future cognitive growth.

One of the most remarkable features of the developing brain is its neuroplasticity—the brain's ability to change and adapt in response to experiences. Neuroplasticity allows the brain to form new connections, strengthen existing ones, and even reorganize itself to compensate for injury or loss of function. This capacity for change is particularly pronounced during early childhood, when the brain is undergoing rapid growth and development.

Neuroplasticity plays a key role in learning. Every time a child learns a new skill or acquires new knowledge, their brain undergoes physical changes. Neurons that are activated during learning form new synapses, and repeated use of these synapses strengthens the connections between neurons. This process is often referred to as "neurons that fire together, wire together." The more a child practices a skill—whether it's learning to speak, ride a bike, or solve a puzzle—the stronger the neural connections related to that skill become.

The brain's plasticity also allows it to recover from injury or adapt to changes in the environment. For example, if a child experiences damage to one area of the brain, other areas may take over the lost function. This phenomenon is particularly evident in cases where children who have had brain injuries early in life are able to recover more fully than adults with similar injuries. The younger the brain, the more plastic it is, making early childhood a time of both vulnerability and opportunity.

Neuroplasticity is not limited to the early years of life, but it is most pronounced during childhood. As the brain matures, it becomes less plastic, meaning that learning new skills and adapting to changes becomes more difficult. However, the brain retains some degree of plasticity throughout life, allowing for continued learning and adaptation.

Enhancing brain development through stimulation is a key way to support cognitive growth in young children. The brain thrives on stimulation, and providing children with a rich and varied environment can help promote the formation of new synapses and the strengthening of existing connections. Stimulation comes in many forms, including sensory experiences, social interactions, physical activity, and intellectual challenges.

Sensory experiences play a fundamental role in brain development. Babies and young children learn about the world through their senses—touch, sight, hearing, taste, and smell. Providing children with a variety of sensory experiences, such as playing with different textures, listening to music, and exploring new environments, helps stimulate the brain and encourages the formation of neural connections. For example, when a baby touches a soft toy or hears a new sound, their brain processes that information and forms connections related to those experiences.

Social interactions are another important form of stimulation for brain development. Children learn from interacting with others, and social experiences help develop cognitive, emotional, and language skills. Talking, reading, and singing to children from an early age stimulates language development and helps build the neural pathways involved in communication. Additionally, play with peers and caregivers promotes problem-solving, cooperation, and emotional regulation—skills that are essential for cognitive development.

Physical activity is also crucial for brain development. Movement and exercise stimulate the brain by increasing blood flow, oxygen, and nutrients to brain cells. Activities such as crawling, walking, running, and climbing help develop motor skills, spatial awareness, and coordination. In addition, physical play encourages the development of executive function skills, such as self-control and planning, by requiring children to navigate rules, take turns, and think ahead.

Intellectual challenges, such as puzzles, games, and problem-solving activities, stimulate the brain by encouraging children to think critically and apply logic. These activities help develop executive function skills, such as working memory, flexible thinking, and self-regulation. For example, when a child works on a puzzle, they must remember where each piece fits, try different strategies, and adjust their approach if their initial attempt doesn't work. These cognitive exercises help strengthen the brain's capacity for learning and adaptation.

One of the most effective ways to enhance brain development through stimulation is by engaging children in play. Play is not only enjoyable but also essential for cognitive growth. Through play, children learn to explore, experiment, and problem-solve in a safe and supportive environment. Play-based learning allows children to develop creativity, curiosity, and critical thinking skills, all of which are essential for cognitive development.

For example, pretend play helps children develop symbolic thinking, as they use objects to represent something else—a block becomes a car, or a stick becomes a sword. This type of play encourages imagination and cognitive flexibility, as children learn to think beyond the concrete and explore abstract ideas. Similarly, building with blocks or playing with puzzles helps children develop spatial awareness, problem-solving skills, and logical thinking. These activities encourage children to think critically about how pieces fit together, how structures can be built, and how to solve challenges they encounter during play.

Another important aspect of enhancing brain development through stimulation is creating a language-rich environment. Language exposure is one of the most powerful stimulants for brain development, particularly in the early years. Talking, reading, and singing to children from birth not only helps them acquire language skills but also supports cognitive processes such as memory, attention, and reasoning. The more words children are exposed to in their early years, the stronger their language and cognitive skills will be later in life. Research has shown that children who are regularly spoken to and engaged in conversation have larger vocabularies and better reading comprehension skills by the time they enter school.

Reading books with children is a particularly effective way to enhance brain development. Reading exposes children to new vocabulary, introduces them to the structure of stories, and stimulates their imagination. It also encourages children to think critically, as they predict what might happen next in a story or relate the events in the book to their own experiences. Furthermore, the interaction between the child and the adult during reading—discussing the story, asking questions, and pointing out details—enhances language development and strengthens the bonds that support emotional growth.

Singing and listening to music also have profound effects on brain development. Music stimulates multiple areas of the brain, including those responsible for language, memory, and motor skills. Songs with repetitive patterns, rhymes, and rhythms help children learn language structures and improve auditory processing. Music also fosters creativity and emotional expression, allowing children to explore sounds, patterns, and movement in a joyful and engaging way.

Creating a stimulating environment for young children goes beyond just providing toys and activities; it involves fostering an environment that encourages curiosity, exploration, and a sense of security. A child's sense of safety and emotional well-being is closely tied to their cognitive development. When children feel secure and loved, their brains are more open to learning and exploring. This is why responsive care-giving—where caregivers are attentive, nurturing, and responsive to a child's needs—is so critical for cognitive and emotional development.

Responsive care-giving creates a secure attachment between the child and the caregiver, which provides the foundation for healthy brain development. A child who feels secure in their relationship with their caregiver is more likely to explore their environment, try new things, and take risks in learning. This sense of security is essential for building confidence and resilience, both of which are important for cognitive development. When children are stressed or anxious, their brain's capacity to learn is diminished, as stress hormones like cortisol can interfere with the brain's ability to form and strengthen neural connections.

In addition to emotional security, a stimulating environment should also provide opportunities for children to encounter novelty and challenge. New experiences, such as visiting new places, meeting new people, or trying new activities, stimulate brain development by encouraging children to adapt to new situations and apply what they've learned to unfamiliar contexts. These novel experiences help build cognitive flexibility, which is the ability to adjust thinking and behavior in response to changing demands or environments—a crucial skill for problem-solving and learning.

Providing appropriate challenges for children is also key to enhancing brain development. When children are given tasks that are just beyond their current abilities, they are encouraged to stretch their cognitive capacities. This is where the concept of the "zone of proximal development," introduced by Vygotsky, becomes relevant. The zone of proximal development refers to the range of tasks that a child can complete with the assistance of a more knowledgeable individual, such as a caregiver, teacher, or peer. By providing support and guidance, adults can help children achieve tasks that they wouldn't be able to accomplish on their own, which fosters cognitive growth.

For example, a child may be able to complete a simple puzzle on their own, but with the help of an adult, they may be able to tackle a more complex puzzle that requires them to think critically and apply new strategies. As the child becomes more proficient, they will be able to complete increasingly difficult tasks independently. This process of scaffolding—where the adult provides just enough support to help the child succeed, then gradually withdraws that support as the child becomes more capable—is a powerful way to enhance brain development through stimulation.

Technology, when used appropriately, can also be a tool for enhancing brain development. Interactive educational apps, games, and programs designed for young children can stimulate cognitive development by providing engaging, hands-on learning experiences. These technologies can reinforce skills such as problem-solving, memory, and language acquisition, especially when they are used in moderation and in conjunction with other forms of learning. However, it is important for caregivers to ensure that screen time is balanced with physical activity, social interaction, and other types of play, as excessive screen time can have negative effects on brain development.

Another crucial element in enhancing brain development is providing opportunities for physical activity. Physical movement stimulates the brain by increasing blood flow and oxygenation, which supports the growth and development of neurons. Activities that involve coordination, balance, and fine motor skills—such as running, jumping, drawing, and manipulating small objects—help strengthen the connections between the brain and the body, fostering the development of both cognitive and motor skills.

Physical activity is particularly important for the development of the cerebellum, the part of the brain responsible for motor control, balance, and coordination. Research has shown that physical activity not only improves motor skills but also enhances cognitive functions such as attention, memory, and problem-solving. Activities like climbing, playing catch, and riding a bike challenge children to think about spatial relationships, timing, and sequencing, all of which contribute to cognitive growth.

Incorporating physical activity into daily routines is an excellent way to support both brain and body development. Outdoor play, in particular, provides children with opportunities to explore their environment, use their imagination, and engage in physical challenges that stimulate their brains. Whether it's running through a park, climbing on a jungle gym, or playing a game of tag, these activities help children build the neural connections that support cognitive, emotional, and social development.

In addition to direct experiences, another way to enhance brain development is by encouraging children to engage in creative and imaginative play. Creative activities such as drawing, painting, building, and role-playing help children develop cognitive flexibility, problem-solving skills, and the ability to think symbolically. When children engage in pretend play, they use their imagination to create scenarios, solve problems, and explore different perspectives. This type of play fosters cognitive growth by encouraging children to think abstractly and experiment with new ideas.

For example, when a child pretends to be a doctor treating a patient, they are not only using their imagination but also practicing problem-solving, decision-making, and empathy. Creative play allows children to explore different roles, experiment with cause-and-effect relationships, and develop a deeper understanding of the world around them. These cognitive processes are essential for developing critical thinking skills that will serve children throughout their lives.

In conclusion, enhancing brain development through stimulation is a multifaceted process that involves providing children with a wide range of experiences, challenges, and opportunities for learning. Whether through sensory experiences, social interactions, physical activity, or creative play, children's brains thrive when they are exposed to rich and varied stimuli. By creating an environment that fosters curiosity, exploration, and emotional security, caregivers and educators can support the formation of strong neural connections that will serve as the foundation for lifelong learning and cognitive growth.

The developing brain is a remarkable organ that responds dynamically to the experiences and environments in which a child is placed. With proper stimulation and support, children's cognitive abilities can flourish, setting the stage for future success in school, relationships, and personal growth. As we continue to learn more about how the brain develops, it becomes increasingly clear that the early years are a critical time for shaping a child's intellectual and emotional capacities, making the role of parents, caregivers, and educators all the more important in nurturing a child's full potential.

The Importance of Play in Cognitive Growth

Play is an integral part of a child's cognitive growth and overall development. It is through play that children engage with the world around them, learn new concepts, develop skills, and form their understanding of how things work. Cognitive growth, which refers to the development of thinking, reasoning, problem-solving, and understanding, is greatly enhanced through play. Children's brains are highly plastic during early childhood, and the experiences they have through different types of play stimulate neural connections that are vital for learning.

Play is not just about having fun; it's a serious business for a child's brain. Various types of play contribute differently to cognitive development, each providing unique benefits that help children master the skills needed for academic success, emotional regulation, and social interaction. As we explore the different types of play, it becomes clear that play is a dynamic and multifaceted activity that supports cognitive growth in a wide range of areas.

There are several types of play that children engage in, each serving distinct purposes in their cognitive development. Broadly, play can be classified into three categories: free play, guided play, and structured play. While these categories overlap, each offers different learning experiences that contribute to a child's cognitive, social, and emotional development.

Free play, often referred to as unstructured or child-led play, is play that is initiated and controlled by the child. In free play, children decide what they want to do, how they want to do it, and when they want to change the activity. This type of play is open-ended and allows for creativity, exploration, and problem-solving without adult interference. Examples of free play include building with blocks, playing dress-up, or running around outside. Free play is crucial for cognitive growth because it allows children to experiment, test out ideas, and make their own decisions. It also promotes self-regulation and autonomy, as children learn to manage their own actions and impulses.

In free play, children engage in problem-solving activities that challenge their thinking and encourage cognitive flexibility. For example, when building with blocks, a child might experiment with different ways to stack them to create a tall tower. If the tower falls, the child must figure out how to balance the blocks better or try a new strategy. This process of trial and error is essential for cognitive development, as it helps children develop critical thinking skills and resilience in the face of challenges.

Guided play, in contrast, is play that is child-led but scaffolded by an adult or more knowledgeable peer. In guided play, the adult sets up an environment or activity that encourages exploration and learning, but the child still has control over their actions and decisions. For example, a parent might set up a toy farm with animals and encourage the child to arrange the animals by type or size, asking open-ended questions to prompt thinking. Guided play strikes a balance between free play and structured learning, allowing children to engage in meaningful exploration while receiving support that helps deepen their understanding of concepts.

One of the key benefits of guided play is that it allows adults to introduce new vocabulary, concepts, and ideas in a natural and engaging way. For instance, while playing with toy animals, a parent might introduce new words such as "herbivore" or "carnivore," expanding the child's language and understanding of the natural world. By guiding the play, adults can ensure that children are exposed to educational content in a fun and interactive way, helping them make connections between what they are playing and the real world.

Structured play, on the other hand, refers to play that is organized and often has specific rules or objectives. This type of play is typically adult-directed and may include games, sports, or educational activities. Examples of structured play include board games, puzzles, team sports, or classroom activities like matching games or memory tasks. Structured play is particularly valuable for teaching specific skills, such as following directions, working collaboratively with others, and developing fine motor skills.

Structured play offers children the opportunity to practice cognitive skills like memory, attention, and logical reasoning. For example, in a game of "Simon Says," children must listen carefully, remember the rules, and inhibit their impulses in order to succeed. These cognitive tasks help strengthen executive function, which includes the skills needed for self-control, planning, and decision-making. Structured play also introduces children to the concept of rules, which is important for developing an understanding of social norms and cooperation.

The balance between free play, guided play, and structured play is essential for fostering cognitive growth. While free play promotes creativity and autonomy, guided play helps scaffold learning by providing support and introducing new concepts. Structured play, meanwhile, offers the opportunity to practice specific cognitive skills in a more controlled environment. Together, these types of play provide a well-rounded foundation for cognitive development, allowing children to learn in diverse and meaningful ways.

In addition to its cognitive benefits, play also has significant social and emotional benefits. Through play, children learn how to interact with others, manage their emotions, and develop a sense of empathy and cooperation. These social and emotional skills are closely linked to cognitive growth, as they enable children to navigate complex social situations and solve problems collaboratively.

During play, children often engage in activities that require negotiation, sharing, and turn-taking, all of which are important for social development. For example, when playing with others, a child may need to negotiate who gets to use a particular toy or decide how to divide roles in a pretend play scenario. These interactions teach children how to communicate their needs, listen to others, and resolve conflicts—skills that are essential for forming positive relationships with peers.

Play also provides a safe space for children to explore their emotions and learn how to manage them. For instance, in pretend play, children may take on different roles and act out scenarios that allow them to express their feelings and work through challenges. A child might pretend to be a superhero to cope with feelings of powerlessness or play house to process family dynamics. This type of play helps children develop emotional regulation skills, as they learn to identify and manage their emotions in a healthy and constructive way.

Furthermore, play fosters empathy and perspective-taking, as children often put themselves in the shoes of others during role-play. For example, when playing "doctor" and "patient," children must think about how the patient feels and what the doctor needs to do to help them. This ability to take on different roles and perspectives is a key component of social-emotional development and contributes to cognitive skills such as theory of mind—the understanding that others have thoughts, feelings, and perspectives that may differ from one's own.

The social and emotional benefits of play are not limited to interactions with peers; they also extend to relationships with caregivers and adults. Play provides an opportunity for bonding and building trust, as caregivers engage in activities that are fun and enjoyable for the child. Whether it's playing a game, reading a story, or engaging in pretend play, these shared experiences strengthen the child's emotional connection to the caregiver, creating a secure base from which the child can explore and learn.

Play-based learning is a powerful strategy for promoting cognitive development in young children. Play-based learning involves using play as a vehicle for teaching academic concepts and cognitive skills in a way that is engaging, interactive, and meaningful for the child. Research has shown that children learn best when they are actively involved in the learning process, and play provides a natural and enjoyable way for them to engage with new concepts.

One of the key elements of play-based learning is that it is child-centered. This means that the learning activities are designed to be relevant and interesting to the child, allowing them to take the lead in their own learning. For example, rather than sitting at a desk and completing a worksheet, a child might engage in a hands-on activity like sorting objects by color or size, counting blocks, or building a structure to explore concepts like math, science, and spatial reasoning. These types of activities allow children to learn through exploration, experimentation, and discovery.

Play-based learning also supports the development of problem-solving and critical thinking skills. When children engage in play, they are often faced with challenges or obstacles that require them to think creatively and come up with solutions. For example, when building a tower with blocks, a child may need to figure out how to balance the blocks to prevent the tower from falling. This process of trial and error helps children develop cognitive flexibility and resilience, as they learn to approach problems from different angles and persist in the face of failure.

Another important aspect of play-based learning is that it encourages collaboration and social interaction. Many play-based activities are designed to be done in groups, allowing children to work together to solve problems, share ideas, and learn from one another. For example, a group of children might work together to build a fort or complete a puzzle, learning valuable skills such as communication, teamwork, and negotiation in the process. These social interactions also support cognitive development, as children learn to consider different perspectives and ideas, enhancing their ability to think critically and solve problems collaboratively.

Play-based learning is also particularly effective for developing early literacy and numeracy skills. For example, through play, children can explore concepts like counting, sorting, and measuring in a hands-on, meaningful way. Activities such as playing shop, where children "buy" and "sell" items, introduce basic math concepts like addition and subtraction. Similarly, pretend play that involves writing lists, signs, or notes helps children develop early writing and reading skills in a context that feels natural and fun.

Language development is another area where play-based learning shines. Through play, children are exposed to new vocabulary and language structures as they engage in conversations with peers and adults. For example, when playing house, children may use words related to cooking, cleaning, and family roles, expanding their vocabulary in a context that is relevant and meaningful to them. Additionally, play provides opportunities for children to practice using language to express their thoughts, ask questions, and solve problems, all of which contribute to their cognitive development.

One of the most significant forms of play for cognitive growth is imaginative and creative play. Imaginative play, also known as pretend play or make-believe play, involves children using their imagination to create scenarios, roles, and narratives that are not tied to their immediate reality. This type of play is often seen when children engage in activities such as pretending to be a superhero, running a pretend grocery store, or taking care of a stuffed animal as if it were a real pet. Imaginative play is a powerful tool for cognitive development because it allows children to explore complex concepts, experiment with different roles, and practice problem-solving in a safe and controlled environment.

One of the key cognitive benefits of imaginative play is that it encourages symbolic thinking. Symbolic thinking is the ability to understand that one thing can represent another, which is a fundamental cognitive skill that underpins language, mathematics, and abstract reasoning. For example, when a child pretends that a block is a phone, they are using that object to symbolically represent something else. This ability to think symbolically is essential for later academic success, as it is the foundation for understanding symbols like letters and numbers.

Imaginative play also fosters creativity and innovation. When children engage in pretend play, they must come up with scenarios, roles, and solutions that are not present in their immediate environment. This type of thinking requires them to use their creativity to imagine new possibilities and explore different ways of thinking. For example, a child who is playing "doctor" might come up with creative ways to "treat" their patient, using toys or household items in new and innovative ways. This type of play helps children develop cognitive flexibility, which is the ability to adapt their thinking and behavior to different situations and challenges.

Imaginative play also supports the development of executive function skills, such as planning, self-regulation, and working memory. When children engage in pretend play, they often create elaborate stories or scenarios that require them to remember details, plan ahead, and follow through on their ideas. For example, if a child is pretending to run a grocery store, they might need to plan what items to sell, organize the "store," and remember the roles that their playmates are playing. These activities help strengthen their working memory and their ability to plan and execute tasks, which are essential skills for academic success.

In addition to its cognitive benefits, imaginative play also has significant social and emotional benefits. Through pretend play, children learn to understand different perspectives and emotions. For example, when a child pretends to be a teacher or a parent, they must think about how that role behaves and what responsibilities it entails. This helps children develop empathy and perspective-taking, as they learn to consider the thoughts and feelings of others. These social-emotional skills are closely linked to cognitive development, as they help children navigate complex social interactions and develop problem-solving skills in collaborative settings.

Creative play, which often overlaps with imaginative play, involves activities such as drawing, painting, building, and crafting. Creative play allows children to express themselves and experiment with different materials, ideas, and techniques. This type of play is crucial for cognitive development because it encourages children to think critically, explore new possibilities, and solve problems in innovative ways. For example, when a child is building a tower with blocks or creating a piece of artwork, they must think about how to arrange the materials, how to overcome obstacles (such as a tower that keeps falling), and how to achieve their desired outcome.

Creative play also supports the development of fine motor skills, which are essential for tasks such as writing, drawing, and using tools. Activities like cutting with scissors, painting with a brush, or building with small blocks help children develop hand-eye coordination and control over their movements. These skills are not only important for artistic expression but also for academic tasks like writing and manipulating objects in science experiments.

Furthermore, creative play fosters a growth mindset, which is the belief that abilities can be developed through effort and practice. When children engage in creative activities, they often face challenges or setbacks, such as a drawing that doesn't turn out the way they envisioned or a block tower that collapses. By persevering through these challenges and experimenting with different approaches, children learn that they can improve their skills and achieve their goals through effort and creativity. This growth mindset is essential for cognitive development, as it encourages children to embrace challenges, persist in the face of difficulties, and approach learning with curiosity and resilience.

In summary, imaginative and creative play are fundamental components of cognitive development. They encourage children to think symbolically, develop creativity, and practice problem-solving skills. These types of play also support the development of executive function skills, such as planning, working memory, and self-regulation, which are critical for academic success. Additionally, imaginative and creative play foster social-emotional skills, such as empathy, perspective-taking, and collaboration, all of which are closely linked to cognitive growth.

The importance of play in cognitive development cannot be overstated. Through different types of play—whether it's free play, guided play, structured play, or imaginative play—children develop the cognitive, social, and emotional skills they need to succeed in school and in life. Play is a natural and enjoyable way for children to explore their world, experiment with new ideas, and develop the skills they need to become confident and capable learners.

As adults, it is important to recognize the value of play and to provide children with ample opportunities to engage in a variety of play experiences. By creating an environment that encourages exploration, creativity, and problem-solving, we can support children's cognitive development and help them reach their full potential. Play is not just a break from learning—it is a vital part of how children learn, grow, and develop the skills they need to navigate the world around them.

Language and Communication Development

Language and communication development is one of the most crucial aspects of early childhood cognitive growth, shaping not only how children interact with the world but also how they think, learn, and process information. From the moment a child is born, language begins to form the foundation of their cognitive abilities, with early experiences in communication influencing how they perceive and understand their surroundings. As children grow, their language development plays a pivotal role in their ability to engage with others, solve problems, and make sense of the world around them.

Language is deeply intertwined with thought, with many scholars arguing that the development of language fundamentally shapes how we think. The relationship between language and thought is a complex and ongoing area of study in cognitive science, with various theories offering different perspectives on how these two cognitive processes influence each other.

One of the most well-known theories about the relationship between language and thought is the linguistic relativity hypothesis, also known as the Sapir-Whorf hypothesis. This theory posits that the language a person speaks influences how they think and perceive the world. For example, some languages have multiple words for different types of snow, while others have only one word for snow. According to the Sapir-Whorf hypothesis, speakers of the language with multiple words for snow may be more attuned to the different types of snow, leading them to perceive and think about snow in more nuanced ways than speakers of a language with only one word for it.

While the strong version of the linguistic relativity hypothesis—that language determines thought—has been largely discredited, there is evidence to suggest that language does shape certain cognitive processes. For instance, studies have shown that language influences memory, categorization, and even perception of time and space. For young children, the development of language provides them with the tools to categorize objects, events, and experiences, which in turn helps them make sense of their environment and form more complex thoughts.

Language also plays a crucial role in the development of self-regulation and executive function, two key components of cognitive growth. As children learn to use language to express their thoughts, desires, and emotions, they also develop the ability to regulate their behavior and make decisions. For example, a child who can articulate that they are feeling frustrated is better able to manage their emotions than a child who lacks the language skills to identify and express their feelings. This ability to use language for self-regulation is an essential skill that supports cognitive development, as it enables children to focus on tasks, solve problems, and navigate social interactions.

The power of talking, reading, and storytelling in supporting language and cognitive development cannot be overstated. From the earliest days of life, infants begin to learn language through exposure to the sounds and rhythms of speech. Even before they can speak, babies are actively listening and absorbing the language around them, laying the groundwork for later language acquisition.

Talking to children from birth is one of the most effective ways to support their language development. When caregivers talk to infants, they are not only providing linguistic input but also fostering social-emotional connections that are essential for cognitive growth. Research has shown that the quantity and quality of language that children are exposed to in the early years have a significant impact on their language development and overall cognitive abilities. Children who are spoken to frequently and engaged in conversations tend to develop larger vocabularies, better listening skills, and stronger language comprehension compared to children who are exposed to less verbal interaction.

Reading to children is another powerful tool for language development. Books expose children to a wide range of vocabulary, sentence structures, and ideas that they might not encounter in everyday conversation. Story-time offers children the opportunity to hear rich and varied language, which helps build their vocabulary and comprehension skills. Furthermore, reading books aloud encourages children to use their imagination and engage with stories on a deeper cognitive level, which supports the development of abstract thinking and problem-solving skills.

In addition to language exposure, the act of reading itself helps children develop important cognitive skills such as attention, memory, and sequencing. When children listen to a story, they must remember the sequence of events, pay attention to the characters and plot, and make predictions about what might happen next. These cognitive tasks help strengthen their executive function, which is critical for academic success and lifelong learning.

Storytelling, in particular, plays a unique role in language and cognitive development. Unlike reading from a book, storytelling involves the creation of narratives from memory or imagination, which encourages children to actively engage with the story and participate in its unfolding. Storytelling allows for more interaction between the storyteller and the child, as the child can ask questions, make suggestions, and even contribute to the story. This type of interaction fosters language development by encouraging children to use their own language skills to communicate their ideas and thoughts.

Storytelling also supports the development of narrative skills, which are essential for understanding and producing coherent stories. Narrative skills are important for academic success, as they form the basis for reading comprehension and writing abilities. Children who are exposed to storytelling from an early age are more likely to develop strong narrative skills, which in turn supports their overall cognitive development.

Bilingualism, or the ability to speak and understand two languages, has a profound impact on cognitive development. While there was once a belief that learning two languages at a young age might confuse children or delay language development, research has shown that bilingualism offers significant cognitive benefits. In fact, children who grow up speaking two languages often outperform their monolingual peers in certain cognitive tasks, particularly those related to executive function.

One of the key cognitive benefits of bilingualism is the enhancement of executive function, which includes skills such as attention, working memory, cognitive flexibility, and self-control. Bilingual children must constantly manage two linguistic systems, switching between languages depending on the context and the person they are speaking to. This mental juggling requires a high degree of cognitive flexibility and attention control, as the child must be able to inhibit one language while activating the other. These executive function skills are not only useful for language tasks but also for a wide range of cognitive processes, including problem-solving, multitasking, and decision-making.

Bilingualism has also been shown to improve meta linguistic awareness, which is the ability to think about language as an abstract system. Bilingual children often develop a heightened awareness of the structure and rules of language, as they are exposed to two different linguistic systems. This awareness helps them understand how language works and enables them to more easily learn additional languages later in life. Moreover, bilingual children tend to have a better understanding of the arbitrary nature of linguistic signs—for example, they know that different languages use different words to refer to the same object (e.g., "dog" in English and "perro" in Spanish), which enhances their cognitive flexibility.

Another important benefit of bilingualism is that it fosters greater cultural awareness and empathy. Bilingual children are often exposed to multiple cultures through their languages, which helps them develop a broader perspective and an appreciation for diversity. This exposure to different cultural contexts supports cognitive development by encouraging children to think critically about social norms, values, and traditions, and by fostering an understanding of multiple viewpoints.

While bilingualism offers many cognitive advantages, it is important to note that maintaining proficiency in both languages requires consistent exposure and practice. In some cases, bilingual children may experience a "dominant" language, where one language becomes stronger than the other due to greater exposure or use in daily life. To support balanced bilingualism, caregivers and educators can provide opportunities for children to engage with both languages in meaningful and interactive ways, such as through conversations, reading, and play.

Supporting language growth in children requires intentional effort and a nurturing environment that encourages communication and learning. There are several practical strategies that caregivers and educators can use to foster language development and cognitive growth.

First and foremost, engaging in frequent and meaningful conversations with children is essential. Caregivers should talk to children from birth, narrating daily activities, asking questions, and encouraging children to express themselves. It is important to use rich and varied language, as children learn new words and concepts by hearing them in context. Open-ended questions, which require more than a yes or no answer, can help stimulate children's thinking and encourage them to use more complex language.

Reading to children regularly is another powerful way to support language development. Caregivers should choose age-appropriate books that introduce new vocabulary and ideas, and they should encourage children to ask questions and engage with the story. Pointing to pictures, discussing characters and events, and predicting what might happen next are all ways to make reading interactive and cognitively stimulating.

Storytelling, as mentioned earlier, is also a valuable tool for language development. Caregivers can create and share stories with children, encouraging them to participate and contribute to the narrative. This interactive approach helps children develop narrative skills and enhances their ability to organize thoughts and ideas.

Another practical tip for supporting language growth is to provide opportunities for social interaction with peers. Children learn language not only from adults but also from interacting with other children. Playmates, group activities, and preschool environments provide rich opportunities for language development as children engage in conversations, negotiate roles in play, and learn to express their ideas and emotions to others.

For bilingual families, it is important to provide consistent exposure to both languages. Caregivers can support bilingualism by speaking their native language at home, reading books in both languages, and encouraging children to watch educational content in both languages. Additionally, creating opportunities for children to interact with native speakers of both languages can help reinforce language proficiency and cultural understanding.

Incorporating music, rhymes, and songs into daily routines is another effective way to support language growth. Children enjoy music, and songs with repetitive patterns, rhymes, and rhythms help them develop phonological awareness, which is critical for reading development. Singing songs together also provides an opportunity for bonding and interaction, further supporting cognitive and emotional growth.

Finally, caregivers should be patient and responsive to children's attempts at communication. It is important to celebrate and encourage every effort a child makes to communicate, whether through gestures, sounds, or words. Providing positive reinforcement and modeling correct language use in a supportive manner helps build children's confidence in their ability to communicate and fosters their motivation to keep trying. When a child mispronounces a word or struggles to articulate a thought, rather than correcting them directly, caregivers can model the correct usage by repeating the word or sentence in a natural and supportive way. This approach allows children to learn without feeling discouraged or embarrassed by their mistakes.

It's also helpful for caregivers to be mindful of their own use of language around children. Speaking clearly, using descriptive language, and expanding on the child's own words can enhance their understanding and vocabulary. For instance, if a child says "big car," a caregiver might respond with, "Yes, that's a very large red car, and it's driving fast down the street." This type of expansion not only confirms the child's statement but also introduces new words and concepts in a meaningful context.

Another practical approach is to incorporate language-building activities into daily routines. Everyday moments, such as preparing meals, getting dressed, or going for a walk, offer opportunities for rich language interactions. Caregivers can describe what they are doing, ask children to participate in conversations about their environment, or encourage them to express their preferences and thoughts. For example, during a trip to the grocery store, a caregiver might ask the child to help identify different fruits and vegetables, talk about their colors and shapes, or discuss what they will be used for when cooking. These interactions help children connect language to real-world experiences, making learning more relevant and engaging.

In settings where multiple caregivers or educators are involved, consistency in language support is important. It can be helpful for all adults in a child's life to be aware of the child's language development goals and to work together to create a supportive environment. This might involve coordinating between parents, teachers, and other caregivers to ensure that the child is receiving ample opportunities for language-rich interactions across different contexts.

In preschool or daycare settings, structured activities that focus on language development, such as circle time, storytelling, and group discussions, can be very effective. Educators can use these opportunities to introduce new vocabulary, encourage children to express their thoughts and ideas, and model good communication skills. In addition, providing access to a variety of books, games, and activities that promote language learning can enhance children's exposure to new words and concepts.

Technology can also play a role in supporting language development, but it should be used thoughtfully and in moderation. Educational apps, videos, and games that focus on language skills can be beneficial when used as part of a balanced approach that includes plenty of face-to-face interaction and play. It's important to ensure that digital content is age-appropriate, engaging, and interactive, and that caregivers are actively involved in guiding the child's use of technology. For example, watching a video together and discussing the content afterward can turn a passive experience into an interactive learning opportunity.

Bilingual families face unique challenges and opportunities when it comes to language development, but with the right strategies, bilingualism can be a significant advantage. One common concern for parents raising bilingual children is language mixing, where a child might use words from both languages in the same sentence. This is a normal part of bilingual language development and is not a sign of confusion. In fact, language mixing often reflects a high level of cognitive flexibility, as the child is able to navigate between two linguistic systems.

To support bilingual language development, it's important to provide consistent exposure to both languages. One common strategy is the "one person, one language" approach, where each caregiver consistently speaks one language to the child. For example, a parent who is fluent in Spanish might speak only Spanish to the child, while the other parent, fluent in English, speaks only English. This approach helps the child associate each language with a specific person, making it easier for them to differentiate between the two languages.

Another strategy is to create a language-rich environment that includes both languages. This can involve reading books in both languages, watching educational programs or videos in both languages, and encouraging the child to engage in conversations with native speakers of each language. Bilingual playgroups or language classes can also provide opportunities for children to practice both languages in a social setting.

It's important to remember that language development varies from child to child, and bilingual children may take slightly longer to reach certain language milestones compared to their monolingual peers. However, this slight delay is temporary, and the long-term cognitive benefits of bilingualism far outweigh any initial challenges. With patience, consistency, and a supportive environment, bilingual children can develop strong language skills in both languages, along with the cognitive flexibility and cultural awareness that bilingualism provides.

In addition to these practical tips, it's important for caregivers and educators to be aware of potential challenges that can affect language development, such as hearing impairments, speech delays, or developmental disorders like autism spectrum disorder (ASD). Early identification and intervention are crucial for addressing these challenges and ensuring that children receive the support they need to develop strong language and communication skills.

If a caregiver or educator notices that a child is not meeting typical language milestones, it's important to seek guidance from a pediatrician, speech-language pathologist, or other specialists. Early intervention services, such as speech therapy or language development programs, can make a significant difference in helping children overcome language delays and reach their full potential.

In conclusion, language and communication development are foundational to cognitive growth, shaping how children think, learn, and interact with the world. The relationship between language and thought is deeply intertwined, with language providing the tools for children to categorize, understand, and express their ideas. Talking, reading, and storytelling are powerful methods for supporting language growth, as they expose children to new vocabulary, sentence structures, and concepts, while also fostering social-emotional connections and cognitive skills.

Bilingualism, far from being a source of confusion, offers significant cognitive benefits, enhancing executive function, cognitive flexibility, and cultural awareness. By providing consistent exposure to both languages and creating opportunities for meaningful interactions, caregivers can support the development of strong language skills in bilingual children.

Ultimately, the key to fostering language and communication development lies in creating a rich and engaging environment where children feel encouraged to express themselves, explore new ideas, and build on their natural curiosity. Whether through conversations, reading, storytelling, or bilingual experiences, caregivers and educators play a vital role in nurturing the language skills that form the foundation for lifelong learning and cognitive growth.

The Role of Parental Engagement

Parental engagement plays a pivotal role in shaping a child's cognitive development, influencing their thinking abilities, emotional well-being, and overall learning experience. The interactions that take place between a parent and child are not merely exchanges of words or actions but serve as the foundation for the child's intellectual and emotional growth. By fostering a supportive, nurturing, and intellectually stimulating environment, parents can significantly enhance their child's ability to think critically, solve problems, and navigate social and academic challenges.

The impact of parent-child interactions on thinking skills is profound and far-reaching. From the earliest stages of life, children learn how to interpret the world around them through their interactions with their parents or primary caregivers. Parents serve as the first and most important teachers, offering not only knowledge but also the emotional security necessary for a child to explore and engage with their environment.

One of the key ways in which parent-child interactions influence thinking skills is through the process of modeling. Children observe and imitate the behavior, language, and problem-solving strategies of their parents. When parents engage in activities that require critical thinking, such as reading, solving puzzles, or discussing complex ideas, children are exposed to these cognitive processes and begin to internalize them. For example, when a parent talks through a problem out loud, explaining their thought process as they make decisions, the child learns how to approach problem-solving in a structured way. This kind of modeling helps children develop the cognitive skills needed for critical thinking and reasoning.

Moreover, the types of conversations that parents have with their children also play a crucial role in cognitive development. Engaging children in meaningful, open-ended conversations encourages them to think critically and express their ideas. When parents ask questions that require more than a simple "yes" or "no" response, they prompt their children to reflect, analyze, and articulate their thoughts. For instance, asking a child, "What do you think will happen next in the story?" or "Why do you think that character made that choice?" encourages the child to engage in higher-order thinking, such as prediction and inference. These cognitive processes are essential for developing problem-solving skills and logical reasoning.

Parent-child interactions also contribute to the development of executive function, which includes skills such as working memory, cognitive flexibility, and self-control. When parents engage children in activities that require planning, decision-making, and the regulation of emotions, they help strengthen these executive function skills. For example, playing a game that involves taking turns, following rules, and adjusting strategies based on new information provides a fun and interactive way for children to practice these important cognitive abilities. Over time, these interactions help children develop the self-regulation and attention skills that are critical for academic success and lifelong learning.

Another important aspect of parental engagement in cognitive development is the provision of a language-rich environment. Parents who talk to their children frequently, read aloud, and expose them to a wide range of vocabulary provide the tools necessary for developing strong language skills. Language is closely tied to cognitive development, as it allows children to organize their thoughts, express their ideas, and engage in abstract reasoning. By engaging in conversations, reading books, and storytelling, parents can help their children build the linguistic foundation that supports cognitive growth.

The importance of emotional support and consistency in parenting cannot be overstated when it comes to cognitive development. Children thrive in environments where they feel safe, loved, and supported, and these emotional conditions are critical for healthy brain development. Emotional security allows children to explore their surroundings, take risks in learning, and engage with new experiences without fear of failure or judgment.

Consistent emotional support from parents helps children develop a sense of trust and confidence, which is essential for cognitive development. When children know that their parents are reliable, responsive, and attentive to their needs, they are more likely to engage in activities that challenge their thinking skills. This is because emotional security reduces anxiety and stress, allowing children to focus on learning and problem-solving rather than worrying about whether they are making mistakes or disappointing their parents.

For example, when a child is learning a new skill, such as riding a bike or solving a puzzle, the emotional support they receive from their parents can make the difference between success and frustration. If a parent provides encouragement, praises the child's effort, and offers guidance when needed, the child is more likely to persist in the face of challenges and develop resilience. On the other hand, if a parent is critical, impatient, or disengaged, the child may become discouraged, anxious, or unwilling to try new things, which can hinder cognitive growth.

In addition to providing emotional support, consistency in parenting is crucial for cognitive development. Consistency refers to the predictability of a parent's behavior, responses, and expectations. When children know what to expect from their parents—whether it's the rules of the household, the routines of daily life, or the consequences of their actions—they are better able to develop self-regulation and decision-making skills. Consistent parenting creates a stable environment in which children can learn, experiment, and grow without fear of uncertainty or inconsistency.

For instance, if a parent consistently reinforces rules about screen time, homework, or bedtime, the child learns to regulate their behavior according to these expectations. This consistency helps children develop the executive function skills needed to manage their time, prioritize tasks, and make responsible decisions. Moreover, when parents are consistent in their emotional responses—such as offering comfort when a child is upset or praising effort rather than just results—children learn to trust their parents and develop a sense of emotional stability.

However, it is important to note that consistency in parenting does not mean rigidity. Children benefit from parents who are flexible and responsive to their individual needs, rather than adhering to strict rules or expectations at all times. The key is to provide a balance between structure and flexibility, allowing children to feel secure while also giving them the freedom to explore and learn at their own pace.

Active and engaged parenting is essential for fostering cognitive development, and there are several strategies that parents can use to support their child's learning and thinking skills. One of the most effective strategies is to be present and attentive during everyday interactions. This means actively listening to the child, asking thoughtful questions, and providing feedback that encourages further exploration and thinking. When parents are fully engaged in conversations and activities with their children, they create an environment that promotes curiosity, problem-solving, and critical thinking.

Another important strategy for active parenting is to create opportunities for learning through play. Play is a powerful tool for cognitive development, as it allows children to experiment, make decisions, and solve problems in a fun and low-pressure environment. Parents can support their child's cognitive growth by engaging in interactive play that challenges their thinking skills. For example, building with blocks, playing board games, or working on puzzles together can help children develop spatial reasoning, logic, and executive function skills. These activities also provide opportunities for parents to model problem-solving strategies and encourage their child to think creatively.

Reading together is another valuable strategy for supporting cognitive development. Shared reading not only exposes children to new vocabulary and ideas but also provides an opportunity for parents to engage in meaningful discussions about the content of the book. Asking open-ended questions, making predictions, and encouraging children to express their thoughts about the story helps develop their language and critical thinking skills. Additionally, reading aloud fosters a love of learning and curiosity, which are essential for cognitive growth.

Parents can also support cognitive development by encouraging independence and self-directed learning. This involves giving children the freedom to explore their interests, make decisions, and solve problems on their own, with guidance and support when needed. For example, if a child is working on a craft project or trying to figure out how a toy works, parents can offer suggestions or ask questions that prompt the child to think through the problem, rather than providing the solution right away. Encouraging children to take the lead in their own learning helps build confidence, autonomy, and critical thinking skills.

It is also important for parents to provide a stimulating environment that fosters cognitive development. This includes offering a variety of age-appropriate toys, books, and activities that challenge the child's thinking skills. For example, providing puzzles, building sets, and art supplies encourages children to engage in creative problem-solving and critical thinking. Additionally, exposing children to new experiences, such as visiting museums, exploring nature, or attending cultural events, helps expand their understanding of the world and promotes cognitive flexibility.

Parenting styles play a significant role in shaping a child's cognitive development and learning abilities. Different parenting styles create different environments for learning, and each style has its own set of advantages and challenges. Understanding how different parenting styles impact cognitive development can help parents adopt strategies that support their child's learning and growth.

One of the most widely recognized frameworks for understanding parenting styles is the model developed by psychologist Diana Baumrind, which categorizes parenting into four main styles: authoritative, authoritarian, permissive, and uninvolved. Each of these styles has different implications for a child's cognitive and emotional development.

Authoritative parenting is often considered the most effective parenting style for promoting cognitive development. Authoritative parents are both responsive and demanding—they provide emotional support and guidance while also setting clear expectations and boundaries. In an authoritative household, children are encouraged to express their thoughts and opinions, but they are also expected to follow rules and take responsibility for their actions.

The authoritative parenting style fosters cognitive development by promoting independence, critical thinking, and problem-solving skills. Children raised in authoritative households are given the freedom to explore and make decisions, but they also receive guidance and feedback from their parents. This balance of autonomy and structure helps children develop self-regulation, executive function, and a sense of responsibility. Additionally, authoritative parents often engage in open-ended conversations with their children, encouraging them to think critically and express their ideas.

In contrast, authoritarian parenting is characterized by high demands and low responsiveness. Authoritarian parents set strict rules and expect obedience without question, often using punishment as a means of enforcing discipline.

While this parenting style may lead to well-behaved children, it can have negative effects on cognitive development.

Children raised in authoritarian households may struggle with decision-making, problem-solving, and independent thinking, as they are often discouraged from expressing their opinions or making choices on their own. Instead of being encouraged to explore and think critically, children in authoritarian households may focus more on avoiding punishment and meeting external expectations. This can stifle creativity and reduce the child's confidence in their ability to solve problems independently. Moreover, the lack of emotional support in authoritarian parenting may lead to anxiety and fear of failure, both of which can hinder cognitive development.

Permissive parenting, on the other hand, is characterized by high responsiveness and low demands. Permissive parents are nurturing and loving but often fail to set clear boundaries or expectations for their children's behavior. While children raised in permissive households may have strong emotional bonds with their parents, they may struggle with self-regulation and discipline. Without clear rules or limits, children may have difficulty developing the executive function skills necessary for managing their time, focusing on tasks, and making responsible decisions.

Permissive parenting can impact cognitive development by allowing too much freedom without the necessary structure to support learning. Children may not be challenged to think critically, solve problems, or regulate their behavior, which can lead to difficulties in academic settings where these skills are required. However, the emotional support provided by permissive parents can foster creativity and emotional intelligence, so long as it is paired with opportunities for cognitive challenge and responsibility.

Uninvolved parenting, sometimes referred to as neglectful parenting, is characterized by low responsiveness and low demands. Uninvolved parents may be disengaged or indifferent to their child's emotional and cognitive needs, providing little guidance, support, or structure. Children raised in uninvolved households may experience significant challenges in cognitive development, as they lack both the emotional security and intellectual stimulation necessary for growth.

Without the presence of engaged parents to model problem-solving, offer feedback, or encourage exploration, children in uninvolved households may struggle with self-esteem, academic achievement, and emotional regulation. This parenting style is associated with the poorest outcomes for cognitive development, as children are often left to navigate the world without the support and resources they need to succeed.

Understanding the impact of different parenting styles on cognitive development is crucial for parents who want to create an environment that fosters learning and growth. While each parenting style has its own strengths and weaknesses, the authoritative style is widely regarded as the most effective for promoting cognitive development. By providing both emotional support and intellectual challenge, authoritative parents help their children develop the skills they need to think critically, solve problems, and regulate their behavior.

However, it is important to recognize that no single parenting style is perfect, and many parents may adopt elements of different styles depending on the situation. The key to effective parenting lies in being responsive to the individual needs of the child and creating a balance between structure and flexibility, support and independence. Parents who are attuned to their child's emotional and cognitive needs are better equipped to provide the guidance and opportunities necessary for healthy development.

In conclusion, parental engagement is one of the most influential factors in shaping a child's cognitive development. Through meaningful interactions, emotional support, and consistent parenting practices, parents can foster an environment that encourages critical thinking, problem-solving, and self-regulation. By adopting active and engaged parenting strategies, creating a language-rich environment, and understanding the impact of different parenting styles, parents can provide their children with the tools they need to succeed academically, socially, and emotionally.

Ultimately, the goal of parental engagement is to help children develop into confident, capable, and curious learners who are equipped to navigate the challenges of the world around them. By being present, responsive, and intentional in their parenting practices, parents play a vital role in supporting their child's cognitive growth and lifelong learning.

Nutrition and Cognitive Development

Nutrition plays a foundational role in the development of a child's brain and cognitive abilities, shaping how they think, learn, and process information throughout life. The relationship between diet and cognitive development is particularly critical in the early years, as this is when the brain undergoes rapid growth and transformation. Providing children with the right nutrients during this period can have long-lasting effects on their intellectual capacities, while poor nutrition can have equally lasting negative consequences. The brain, as the body's most energy-demanding organ, requires a steady supply of essential nutrients to fuel its development and functioning.

During infancy and early childhood, the brain grows at an extraordinary rate, requiring a complex array of nutrients to form neurons, synapses, and other critical structures. The first few years of life are a critical period for brain development, as millions of neural connections are formed daily, enabling the child to process sensory input, develop language skills, and engage in problem-solving. Nutritional deficiencies during this time can lead to cognitive delays, impair learning, and hinder emotional regulation. Thus, understanding the essential nutrients necessary for optimal brain development and how diet influences cognitive abilities is crucial for parents, caregivers, and educators.

Several key nutrients are essential for healthy brain development, and their absence or insufficiency can lead to significant developmental issues. The most critical of these nutrients include omega-3 fatty acids, particularly docosahexaenoic acid (DHA), proteins, iron, zinc, iodine, vitamins (such as B vitamins and vitamin D), and antioxidants. Each of these nutrients serves a unique function in brain development and cognitive functioning.

Omega-3 fatty acids, particularly DHA, are among the most important nutrients for brain health. DHA is a structural component of the brain's cell membranes and plays a key role in the development of the cerebral cortex, the part of the brain responsible for memory, language, and higher cognitive functions. DHA also influences the fluidity of cell membranes, which is essential for the transmission of signals between neurons. Studies have shown that DHA is crucial for the development of the retina and visual cortex, enhancing both cognitive and sensory processing abilities. A deficiency in omega-3 fatty acids during critical periods of brain development can result in structural abnormalities in the brain and impairments in cognitive functions such as attention, memory, and learning.

Proteins, often referred to as the building blocks of the body, are equally vital for brain development. Proteins are made up of amino acids, which are necessary for the synthesis of neurotransmitters, the chemicals that transmit signals between neurons. Neurotransmitters such as serotonin, dopamine, and norepinephrine are essential for regulating mood, attention, and cognition. Adequate protein intake ensures that the brain has the necessary amino acids to produce these neurotransmitters and maintain optimal cognitive functioning.

Iron is another essential nutrient for brain development, particularly during infancy and early childhood. Iron is required for the production of hemoglobin, the protein in red blood cells that transports oxygen throughout the body, including to the brain. Oxygen is essential for energy production in brain cells, and a lack of oxygen can impair cognitive functions. Iron is also involved in the synthesis of myelin, the protective coating around neurons that speeds up the transmission of electrical signals. Myelin is crucial for efficient communication between neurons, and a deficiency in iron can slow cognitive processing and hinder learning. Iron-deficiency anemia, a condition in which the body lacks enough iron to produce sufficient hemoglobin, is associated with impaired cognitive development, attention deficits, and poor academic performance.

Zinc is another important nutrient for cognitive development. Zinc plays a role in cellular growth and the regulation of neurotransmitters such as glutamate and GABA, which are essential for learning and memory. Zinc is also involved in synaptic plasticity, the brain's ability to adapt and form new connections in response to learning and experience. A deficiency in zinc can lead to impairments in memory formation, attention, and spatial learning.

Iodine is particularly critical for brain development because it is essential for the production of thyroid hormones, which regulate the growth and development of the brain. Iodine deficiency, particularly during pregnancy and early childhood, can lead to cognitive impairments, developmental delays, and even cretinism, a severe form of intellectual disability. Even mild iodine deficiency has been linked to lower IQ scores and reduced academic performance.

In addition to these nutrients, vitamins also play a crucial role in brain development. B vitamins, including B6, B12, and folate, are necessary for the production of neurotransmitters and for the maintenance of brain health. Folate, in particular, is critical during pregnancy, as it helps prevent neural tube defects and supports the development of the brain and spinal cord. Vitamin D is also important for brain health, as it helps regulate calcium levels in the brain and supports the functioning of neurons. Vitamin D deficiency has been associated with cognitive impairments, mood disorders, and an increased risk of neurodegenerative diseases.

Antioxidants, such as vitamins C and E, play a protective role in brain development by neutralizing free radicals, which can damage brain cells. The developing brain is particularly vulnerable to oxidative stress, which can disrupt the formation of neurons and synapses. Antioxidants help protect the brain from this damage, ensuring that cognitive development proceeds smoothly.

The impact of diet on cognitive abilities is significant, and the quality of a child's diet can influence their intellectual functioning in both the short and long term. A diet that is rich in essential nutrients supports optimal brain development and cognitive functioning, while a diet that is deficient in these nutrients can lead to cognitive impairments and developmental delays.

For example, research has shown that children who consume diets high in saturated fats and refined sugars perform worse on cognitive tasks related to memory, attention, and learning compared to children who consume diets rich in fruits, vegetables, whole grains, and healthy fats. Diets high in processed foods and low in essential nutrients can lead to inflammation in the brain, impairing cognitive functions and increasing the risk of mental health disorders such as anxiety and depression.

On the other hand, a balanced diet that includes a variety of nutrient-dense foods can enhance cognitive abilities and support academic achievement. Studies have shown that children who consume diets rich in fruits, vegetables, whole grains, lean proteins, and healthy fats perform better on tests of cognitive function, have better memory and attention, and are more likely to succeed academically. This is because these foods provide the brain with the necessary nutrients to support neurotransmitter production, synaptic plasticity, and overall brain health.

The foods that boost brain power are those that are rich in essential nutrients such as omega-3 fatty acids, antioxidants, vitamins, and minerals. These foods provide the brain with the building blocks it needs to grow and function effectively, supporting cognitive abilities such as memory, attention, and problem-solving.

Omega-3 fatty acids, particularly DHA and EPA, are found in fatty fish such as salmon, mackerel, sardines, and trout. These fatty acids are critical for brain development and cognitive functioning, and consuming foods rich in omega-3s has been shown to improve memory, attention, and learning. For children who do not consume fish regularly, omega-3 supplements derived from fish oil or algae can be an effective way to ensure adequate intake.

Antioxidant-rich foods, such as berries (blueberries, strawberries, and blackberries), leafy greens (spinach, kale), and nuts (almonds, walnuts), help protect the brain from oxidative stress and inflammation. Berries, in particular, are high in flavonoids, a type of antioxidant that has been shown to improve memory and cognitive function. Leafy greens are also rich in folate and other B vitamins, which support the production of neurotransmitters and help maintain brain health.

Whole grains, such as oats, quinoa, brown rice, and whole wheat, provide a steady supply of glucose, the brain's primary source of energy. Unlike refined carbohydrates, which cause spikes and crashes in blood sugar levels, whole grains release glucose slowly, providing a stable source of energy for the brain and supporting sustained attention and concentration.

Eggs are another excellent food for brain health, as they are rich in choline, a nutrient that is essential for the production of acetylcholine, a neurotransmitter involved in memory and learning. Choline is also important for the development of the brain's hippocampus, the region responsible for memory formation.

Other brain-boosting foods include nuts and seeds, which are high in healthy fats, vitamin E, and antioxidants. Walnuts, in particular, are rich in DHA, while almonds provide vitamin E, which protects the brain from oxidative damage. Seeds such as flaxseeds and chia seeds are excellent sources of plant-based omega-3 fatty acids and can easily be added to smoothies, cereals, or salads.

Lean proteins, such as chicken, turkey, beans, and legumes, provide the amino acids necessary for neurotransmitter production and cognitive functioning. These proteins also help stabilize blood sugar levels, preventing energy crashes that can impair focus and attention.

The role of gut health in cognitive development is an emerging area of research that highlights the connection between the brain and the digestive system, often referred to as the gut-brain axis. The gut is home to trillions of bacteria, collectively known as the gut microbiota, which play a crucial role in digestion, immune function, and even cognitive development.

The gut microbiota produce a variety of compounds that can influence brain function, including neurotransmitters such as serotonin and dopamine. These neurotransmitters are not only involved in mood regulation but also play a key role in cognitive functions such as memory, learning, and attention. An imbalance in the gut microbiota, often caused by poor diet, stress, or antibiotics, can lead to inflammation and disruptions in neurotransmitter production, which can impair cognitive functioning and increase the risk of mental health disorders.

Moreover, the gut microbiota are involved in the production of short-chain fatty acids (SCFAs), which have anti-inflammatory properties and support brain health. SCFAs are produced when dietary fiber is fermented by gut bacteria, and they play a role in maintaining the integrity of the gut barrier, preventing harmful substances from entering the bloodstream and potentially affecting brain function. Research has shown that a healthy, balanced gut microbiota can support cognitive development by promoting a healthy immune system and reducing inflammation, both of which are crucial for brain health.

The relationship between gut health and cognitive development is often referred to as the gut-brain axis, highlighting the bidirectional communication between the gut and the brain. This connection means that what happens in the gut can directly influence brain function and vice versa. For example, stress and anxiety can alter the gut microbiota, leading to gastrointestinal symptoms, while a poor diet can negatively impact both gut health and cognitive abilities.

Maintaining a healthy gut microbiota is essential for supporting brain development and cognitive function, particularly during early childhood when the brain is still developing. A diet rich in fiber, probiotics, and prebiotics can help promote a diverse and healthy gut microbiota, which in turn supports cognitive health.

Probiotics are live beneficial bacteria that can be found in fermented foods such as yogurt, kefir, sauerkraut, kimchi, and miso. These foods help populate the gut with healthy bacteria, supporting digestion, immune function, and brain health. Consuming probiotic-rich foods has been linked to improvements in mood, memory, and cognitive function, as these bacteria produce neurotransmitters and other compounds that influence brain function.

Prebiotics, on the other hand, are types of dietary fiber that serve as food for the beneficial bacteria in the gut. Prebiotics can be found in foods such as garlic, onions, leeks, asparagus, bananas, and whole grains. By feeding the good bacteria in the gut, prebiotics help promote the growth of a healthy microbiota, which supports cognitive development and reduces inflammation in the body.

In addition to promoting a healthy gut through diet, it is important to avoid foods that can negatively impact gut health and, by extension, cognitive function. Diets high in processed foods, sugar, and unhealthy fats can disrupt the balance of gut bacteria, leading to dysbiosis, a condition in which harmful bacteria outnumber beneficial bacteria. Dysbiosis is associated with inflammation, impaired cognitive function, and an increased risk of mental health disorders such as anxiety and depression. Reducing the consumption of processed foods and focusing on whole, nutrient-dense foods can help support both gut health and brain development.

The link between gut health and cognitive development is further supported by research on conditions such as autism spectrum disorder (ASD), attention-deficit/hyperactivity disorder (ADHD), and other neurodevelopmental disorders. Studies have shown that children with these conditions often have altered gut microbiota, and improving gut health through diet and probiotics may help alleviate some of the cognitive and behavioral symptoms associated with these disorders. While more research is needed to fully understand the role of the gut microbiota in neurodevelopmental disorders, the existing evidence suggests that a healthy gut is essential for optimal cognitive development.

In summary, the role of nutrition in cognitive development is multifaceted, involving a complex interplay of essential nutrients, dietary patterns, and gut health. Ensuring that children receive adequate amounts of key nutrients such as omega-3 fatty acids, proteins, iron, zinc, iodine, and vitamins is critical for supporting brain growth, synaptic plasticity, and the production of neurotransmitters. A balanced diet rich in fruits, vegetables, whole grains, lean proteins, and healthy fats provides the brain with the nutrients it needs to function optimally, while diets high in processed foods and sugar can impair cognitive abilities and increase the risk of developmental delays.

Foods that boost brain power, such as fatty fish, leafy greens, berries, nuts, and seeds, are rich in the nutrients needed to support memory, attention, and learning. Incorporating these foods into a child's diet can enhance their cognitive abilities and promote academic success. Additionally, maintaining a healthy gut microbiota through the consumption of probiotics, prebiotics, and fiber-rich foods plays a crucial role in cognitive development by supporting neurotransmitter production, reducing inflammation, and protecting the brain from oxidative stress.

As research on the gut-brain axis continues to grow, it becomes increasingly clear that a holistic approach to nutrition—one that takes into account both the brain and the gut—is essential for fostering cognitive development. By providing children with a nutrient-rich diet and supporting gut health, parents and caregivers can give their children the best possible foundation for cognitive growth and lifelong learning.

The Impact of Early Learning Environments

The early learning environment is one of the most influential factors in a child's cognitive development. It encompasses both the physical and emotional surroundings in which a child grows and learns, starting from their home to educational settings such as daycare and preschool. These environments serve as the foundation for cognitive growth, shaping how children think, solve problems, and acquire new knowledge. Children's brains are highly plastic during the early years, and the quality of their environments has a profound impact on their cognitive abilities. Parents, caregivers, and educators play a critical role in creating nurturing, stimulating, and supportive environments that promote learning and development.

The home is the first and most influential learning environment for a child. From birth, children are immersed in their home environment, and it is here that they begin to make sense of the world around them. The interactions children have with their parents and caregivers, the objects they are exposed to, and the experiences they encounter within the home all contribute to their cognitive development. The home environment sets the stage for early learning by providing children with opportunities to explore, experiment, and engage in activities that stimulate their thinking.

One of the most significant aspects of the home as a learning environment is the role of parent-child interactions. The quality and quantity of these interactions have a direct impact on a child's cognitive development. Children learn language, problem-solving skills, and social norms by observing and interacting with their caregivers. For example, when a parent reads a book to their child, engages in conversation, or encourages exploration, they are providing valuable opportunities for the child to develop cognitive skills such as language comprehension, critical thinking, and memory. These early interactions also foster emotional security, which is essential for learning, as children who feel safe and supported are more likely to engage in new experiences and take intellectual risks.

Additionally, the materials and experiences provided within the home play a critical role in cognitive development. A home rich in learning materials—such as books, puzzles, building blocks, and art supplies—encourages children to engage in activities that promote problem-solving, creativity, and critical thinking. For example, building with blocks helps children develop spatial reasoning skills, while playing with puzzles enhances their ability to think logically and solve problems. These types of activities lay the foundation for more complex cognitive processes that children will use throughout their academic and personal lives.

Another important element of the home environment is the inclusion of routines and consistency. Predictable routines, such as reading before bed or engaging in daily playtime, provide structure and security for young children, which helps them focus on learning. Consistent routines also help children develop executive function skills, such as self-regulation, attention, and planning. For example, knowing that certain tasks or activities happen at specific times each day helps children learn to manage their time and anticipate what comes next, which are important skills for later academic success.

While the home environment provides the foundation for early learning, high-quality early education programs can further support and enhance cognitive development. Research has consistently shown that children who attend high-quality early education programs demonstrate better cognitive outcomes than those who do not. These programs provide children with structured learning experiences, access to educational materials, and opportunities for social interaction, all of which contribute to cognitive growth.

High-quality early education programs are characterized by several key components. First and foremost, these programs provide a rich, stimulating curriculum that is developmentally appropriate and tailored to the needs of young children. The curriculum should include a balance of activities that promote different areas of cognitive development, such as language and literacy, math and reasoning, science exploration, and creative expression. For example, a high-quality program may include story-time to promote language development, hands-on science experiments to encourage inquiry and observation, and art activities to foster creativity and fine motor skills.

Another critical component of high-quality early education programs is the presence of well-trained, responsive educators. Teachers in these programs play a crucial role in facilitating learning by providing guidance, encouragement, and support. They create a warm, nurturing environment that fosters a sense of security and belonging, allowing children to feel comfortable exploring new ideas and taking intellectual risks. Effective educators also engage children in conversations that extend their thinking, ask open-ended questions that encourage critical thinking, and provide opportunities for children to solve problems on their own.

Social interaction is another important element of high-quality early edu-cation programs. These programs provide children with opportunities to interact with their peers in a structured setting, which helps them develop social and emotional skills that are closely linked to cognitive development. For example, working together on group projects or engaging in collaborative play helps children learn how to negotiate, share, and cooperate—skills that are essential for cognitive growth. Additionally, interacting with peers exposes children to new ideas and perspectives, which can enhance their problem-solving abilities and promote cognitive flexibility.

High-quality early education programs also provide children with access to a variety of learning materials and experiences that support cognitive development. For example, classrooms may be equipped with books, educational toys, art supplies, science materials, and technology that encourage exploration and hands-on learning. These materials provide children with the tools they need to engage in creative problem-solving, experiment with new ideas, and develop a deeper understanding of the world around them.

The role of daycare and preschool in cognitive growth is significant, particularly for children whose parents may not have the resources or time to provide a rich learning environment at home. Daycare and preschool programs offer structured, educational experiences that can help bridge the gap between home and formal schooling, providing children with the cognitive and social skills they need to succeed in kindergarten and beyond.

Daycare centers that emphasize early learning through play-based activities and structured curricula can have a positive impact on cognitive development. Play is a natural way for children to explore their environment, experiment with new concepts, and develop problem-solving skills. For example, when children engage in pretend play, they use their imagination to create scenarios, roles, and rules, which fosters cognitive flexibility and creativity. Similarly, when children participate in activities such as building with blocks, solving puzzles, or engaging in sensory play, they develop spatial reasoning, fine motor skills, and critical thinking abilities.

Preschool programs, which are often more structured than daycare, play a critical role in preparing children for formal schooling. These programs introduce children to basic academic concepts, such as letter recognition, counting, and shape identification, while also fostering the development of executive function skills such as attention, memory, and self-regulation. For example, circle time activities, in which children listen to stories, sing songs, and participate in group discussions, help develop their listening skills, language comprehension, and ability to follow directions. These early experiences provide a foundation for the more formal academic learning that will take place in kindergarten and elementary school.

In addition to academic preparation, preschool programs also promote social and emotional development, which is closely linked to cognitive growth. Through interactions with teachers and peers, children learn how to express their emotions, manage conflicts, and work collaboratively with others. These social skills are essential for cognitive development, as they help children navigate complex social situations, think critically about others' perspectives, and develop problem-solving abilities.

Setting up a stimulating home learning space is one of the most effective ways for parents to support their child's cognitive development. A well-designed learning space provides children with access to materials and activities that encourage exploration, creativity, and critical thinking, while also fostering a love of learning. Creating a stimulating learning environment at home does not require a large space or expensive materials—what matters most is that the space is organized, inviting, and tailored to the child's interests and developmental needs.

One of the first steps in setting up a home learning space is to create an environment that is conducive to focused, uninterrupted play and learning. This means choosing a quiet, well-lit area where the child can engage in activities without distractions. For example, a corner of the living room or a dedicated playroom can serve as a learning space, provided it is free from noise, clutter, and distractions such as television or electronic devices.

Once the space has been designated, it's important to stock it with a variety of learning materials that promote cognitive development. These materials should include books, puzzles, building blocks, art supplies, and educational toys that encourage hands-on exploration and problem-solving.

For example, providing children with access to a variety of books fosters language development and critical thinking, while puzzles and building toys enhance spatial reasoning and fine motor skills.

Rotating materials and activities on a regular basis can also help keep the learning space fresh and engaging for children. For example, parents might introduce new puzzles or building sets every few weeks, or swap out art supplies to encourage children to experiment with different materials. By regularly updating the learning space, parents can provide their children with new challenges and opportunities for exploration, which helps support cognitive growth.

In addition to providing materials for structured activities, it's important to include open-ended materials that encourage creativity and imaginative play. For example, items such as cardboard boxes, dress-up clothes, and natural materials (such as stones, sticks, and leaves) allow children to engage in pretend play, which fosters cognitive flexibility and problem-solving. Open-ended materials also encourage children to use their imagination to create their own scenarios, stories, and rules, which enhances their ability to think critically and adapt to new situations.

Another important aspect of a stimulating home learning space is providing opportunities for independent learning. While parent-child interactions are essential for cognitive development, it is equally important for children to have time and space to explore and experiment on their own. A well-designed learning space should encourage independence by making materials accessible and easy to use. For example, storing toys, books, and art supplies on low shelves allows children to choose their own activities and materials, which fosters autonomy and decision-making skills.

Finally, it's important to create a learning space that reflects the child's interests and developmental stage. Parents can tailor the learning environment to their child's individual needs by observing what types of activities and materials engage their child the most. For example, if a child shows a strong interest in animals, the learning space might include books about animals, toy animals for pretend play, and puzzles featuring different species. By aligning the learning space with the child's interests, parents can create an environment that captures the child's curiosity and motivates them to engage in learning activities. This personalization helps the child feel ownership of the space, making them more likely to spend time exploring and engaging in cognitive development tasks that feel enjoyable rather than forced.

In addition to aligning the home learning space with a child's interests, it's essential for parents to recognize the developmental needs of their child at various stages of growth. For younger children, the learning space might focus more on sensory play and motor development, with materials such as stacking toys, blocks, and textured objects. As children grow older and their cognitive abilities expand, the learning space can evolve to include more complex puzzles, science kits, art projects, and books with deeper themes to support their growing curiosity and problem-solving skills.

A stimulating home learning space can also include technology when used thoughtfully and in moderation. Digital tools, such as educational apps or interactive games, can supplement hands-on learning by offering interactive activities that promote cognitive growth in areas like math, language, and reasoning. However, it's important to ensure that technology is balanced with real-world, physical exploration, as excessive screen time can limit opportunities for creative and active play, which are vital for brain development.

Beyond the physical setup, the atmosphere of the learning space is equally important. A positive, nurturing, and supportive environment is critical for fostering a love of learning and intellectual curiosity. Parents can create a welcoming atmosphere by being actively engaged in their child's learning experiences, offering encouragement, and celebrating their child's achievements—whether big or small. This emotional support helps children build the confidence they need to tackle new challenges and persist through difficulties, which are key components of cognitive resilience and growth.

Engaging with children in the learning space also provides parents with valuable opportunities to model thinking processes and problem-solving strategies. For example, when a child is working on a puzzle or building a structure with blocks, parents can offer guidance by asking open-ended questions like, "What do you think would happen if you tried this?" or "How could we make this even taller?" These questions encourage the child to think critically, analyze the situation, and come up with solutions on their own. This type of engagement not only supports cognitive development but also helps children feel capable and empowered as learners.

Incorporating family routines and traditions into the home learning space can also enhance cognitive development. For instance, establishing a regular "family reading time" or "science experiment day" can make learning a natural part of everyday life. These routines create positive associations with learning and provide consistency, which is important for cognitive growth. Children who regularly engage in learning activities as part of their daily routine are more likely to develop lifelong habits of curiosity, exploration, and intellectual engagement.

Furthermore, the integration of outdoor spaces into the home learning environment can expand opportunities for cognitive development. Nature provides an endless array of learning experiences that stimulate curiosity, critical thinking, and problem-solving. Whether it's exploring a backyard, visiting a park, or simply observing the changes in the weather, outdoor learning offers opportunities for children to engage with the natural world and develop a deeper understanding of scientific concepts such as biology, physics, and environmental science.

Outdoor play also encourages physical movement, which has been shown to enhance cognitive function. Activities such as running, climbing, and playing sports help develop spatial awareness, coordination, and executive function skills such as planning and self-regulation. Parents can further enhance outdoor learning by incorporating activities like nature scavenger hunts, gardening, or building simple outdoor projects, all of which promote hands-on problem-solving and exploration.

The emotional climate of the home plays a significant role in how well a child engages with their learning environment. Children need to feel secure, supported, and encouraged in order to explore their learning space with confidence. This emotional safety allows children to take intellectual risks, such as attempting a challenging puzzle or exploring a new concept. When parents provide reassurance and praise effort over outcomes, children learn that making mistakes is part of the learning process and that perseverance leads to success.

For children attending daycare or preschool, parents can enhance cognitive growth by reinforcing what is learned in these settings at home. By maintaining open communication with teachers and caregivers, parents can stay informed about their child's progress and interests and incorporate similar activities into the home learning environment. For example, if a child is learning about shapes in preschool, parents can provide shape-sorting toys or engage in discussions about shapes found in everyday objects at home. This reinforcement helps solidify the child's understanding of key concepts and strengthens the connection between home and school learning.

Similarly, parents can support cognitive development by encouraging self-directed learning. This involves giving children the autonomy to choose activities that interest them and allowing them to explore those activities at their own pace. Providing a variety of materials and options in the learning space encourages children to follow their curiosity and engage deeply with the subject matter that excites them. Self-directed learning promotes independence, critical thinking, and intrinsic motivation, all of which are essential for cognitive development.

It's also important for parents to recognize the value of unstructured play in cognitive growth. While structured activities like reading, puzzles, and educational games are beneficial, unstructured play allows children to use their imagination, explore ideas, and develop creativity. Children who engage in unstructured play are free to create their own scenarios, rules, and challenges, which enhances their problem-solving abilities and cognitive flexibility. For example, a child playing with dolls or action figures might invent a story with complex characters and events, practicing narrative skills and developing an understanding of cause-and-effect relationships in the process.

In addition, parents should encourage a growth mindset in the home learning environment. A growth mindset, as opposed to a fixed mindset, is the belief that intelligence and abilities can be developed through effort and practice. By praising effort and persistence rather than innate talent, parents can help their children develop a positive attitude toward learning and a willingness to tackle challenges. For example, when a child struggles with a difficult puzzle, instead of saying, "You're so smart," parents can say, "I'm proud of how hard you're working to figure this out." This approach teaches children that their abilities are not fixed but can improve with effort, which is critical for fostering a lifelong love of learning and intellectual growth.

Ultimately, the early learning environments that children are exposed to—whether at home, in daycare, or in preschool—play a significant role in shaping their cognitive development. These environments provide the foundation for critical thinking, problem-solving, language acquisition, and social interaction, all of which are essential for academic success and lifelong learning. By creating stimulating, supportive, and engaging learning environments, parents and educators can nurture children's cognitive abilities and help them reach their full intellectual potential.

In conclusion, the early years of a child's life are a critical period for cognitive development, and the environments in which they learn and grow play a central role in shaping their thinking abilities. From the home as the first learning environment to the high-quality early education programs offered by daycare and preschool, children's cognitive development is profoundly influenced by the experiences they have and the support they receive. By setting up stimulating learning spaces, engaging in meaningful interactions, and encouraging self-directed and imaginative play, parents and caregivers can provide children with the tools they need to thrive cognitively, both now and in the future.

The Power of Social Interactions

Social interactions play a fundamental role in shaping a child's cognitive development. Through engagement with peers, siblings, and adults, children learn to navigate complex social dynamics, develop problem-solving skills, and improve their ability to think critically and regulate their emotions. The relationships children build with others are vital for intellectual growth, as socialization is not merely about learning to communicate; it is a powerful tool for expanding cognitive capacities. These interactions offer opportunities for collaboration, negotiation, and conflict resolution, all of which contribute to the development of a child's executive functions, creativity, and overall cognitive abilities.

The role of peers and siblings in cognitive development cannot be understated. While parents and caregivers provide the initial foundation for a child's understanding of the world, peers and siblings introduce a different layer of complexity to social interactions. These relationships are often characterized by equality in status, allowing children to explore new ways of thinking and interacting in a less structured environment compared to adult-child interactions. Peers and siblings often share similar cognitive levels, which makes their interactions particularly effective for learning new skills and solving problems collaboratively.

Siblings, especially, have a unique influence on cognitive development. Older siblings often take on the role of a teacher, modeling behaviors, language, and problem-solving strategies for their younger siblings. This relationship allows for cognitive scaffolding, where the older sibling provides the necessary support for the younger one to engage in more complex tasks than they could manage alone. For instance, when an older sibling helps a younger one complete a puzzle or explains a new game, they are fostering the younger sibling's understanding of spatial relationships, rules, and strategies. Over time, this guidance leads to the younger sibling's cognitive development, as they begin to internalize these problem-solving techniques and apply them independently.

Conversely, younger siblings also contribute to the cognitive development of their older counterparts. By interacting with a younger sibling, the older child learns to simplify complex concepts, break tasks into smaller steps, and practice patience and leadership skills. This process of teaching reinforces the older sibling's understanding of the subject matter and encourages them to think critically about how to convey information clearly and effectively. In this way, the relationship between siblings creates a dynamic learning environment where both parties benefit cognitively from their interactions.

Peers, on the other hand, introduce children to diverse perspectives and problem-solving approaches. Interacting with peers allows children to test the limits of their thinking and adjust their cognitive strategies based on feedback from others. For example, during cooperative play, children must negotiate roles, make decisions, and solve problems together. These experiences require children to consider different viewpoints and adjust their thinking to accommodate the needs and ideas of others. This process not only enhances cognitive flexibility but also promotes the development of social cognition—the ability to understand and interpret the thoughts and intentions of others.

The role of peers in cognitive development is also evident in the concept of peer learning, where children learn from one another through observation, imitation, and collaboration. Peer learning is particularly effective because it allows children to engage in tasks that are slightly beyond their current abilities, a concept known as the zone of proximal development, introduced by psychologist Lev Vygotsky. In this zone, children can accomplish more with the help of a peer or adult than they could on their own. For example, a child who is struggling to understand a math concept may grasp it more easily when a peer explains it in a relatable and accessible way. These peer interactions not only enhance understanding but also boost confidence, as children realize that they are capable of learning new skills with the support of others.

Socialization plays a critical role in the development of problem-solving skills. From a young age, children encounter situations that require them to negotiate, collaborate, and resolve conflicts with others. These social experiences provide valuable opportunities for children to practice problem-solving in real-world contexts, where the solutions are not always straightforward and may require compromise or creative thinking.

During play, children are frequently faced with problems that require social negotiation, such as deciding who will take on which role in a game or figuring out how to share limited resources. These situations force children to think critically about how to balance their own desires with the needs and perspectives of others. For example, in a group of children playing house, one child might want to be the parent while another wants to play the same role. The group must work together to find a solution, whether through taking turns, creating multiple roles, or developing a new game altogether. These problem-solving processes enhance cognitive flexibility and encourage children to think beyond their own immediate desires.

Additionally, social problem-solving requires children to develop and apply executive function skills, such as working memory, inhibitory control, and cognitive flexibility. For example, when two children disagree about how to build a structure with blocks, they must remember each other's ideas, inhibit their own impulses to act immediately, and adapt their thinking to reach a compromise. These cognitive tasks are essential for developing the skills needed to navigate social situations and solve problems in academic and real-life settings.

Moreover, socialization helps children develop the ability to anticipate and understand the emotions and intentions of others, a skill known as theory of mind. Theory of mind allows children to recognize that other people have thoughts, feelings, and perspectives that may differ from their own. This cognitive ability is crucial for effective problem-solving, as it enables children to consider multiple viewpoints and develop solutions that are acceptable to all parties involved. For example, if a child recognizes that their friend is upset about losing a game, they may adjust their behavior to be more supportive, demonstrating both social awareness and cognitive flexibility.

Group play is particularly effective in enhancing executive functioning, which encompasses a range of cognitive processes that are essential for goal-directed behavior, such as planning, attention, problem-solving, and self-regulation. Group play provides a context in which children must apply these skills in dynamic and often unpredictable situations, fostering the development of executive function in a natural and engaging way.

One of the primary ways group play enhances executive functioning is by requiring children to follow rules and work together toward a common goal. For example, in a game of tag, children must regulate their behavior by following the rules of the game (e.g., not stepping out of bounds), monitor their surroundings to avoid being tagged, and plan their movements to stay in the game. These tasks require the use of working memory (remembering the rules and strategy), inhibitory control (resisting the temptation to break the rules), and cognitive flexibility (adapting to changes in the game). Over time, repeated engagement in such activities strengthens these executive function skills, making children more adept at focusing, planning, and problem-solving in both social and academic contexts.

Group play also fosters the development of cooperation and teamwork, which are essential for cognitive growth. When children play together in a group, they must communicate, share resources, and collaborate to achieve a common goal. For example, when building a tower with blocks, children must work together to plan the structure, share materials, and take turns placing blocks. This type of collaborative problem-solving promotes the development of cognitive flexibility, as children learn to adapt their thinking and strategies based on input from others.

Moreover, group play often involves conflict resolution, which provides valuable opportunities for cognitive growth. When conflicts arise during play—such as disagreements over rules or turns—children must use their problem-solving skills to resolve the issue in a way that is fair to everyone involved. These experiences teach children how to negotiate, compromise, and think critically about how to balance different perspectives. Conflict resolution during group play also enhances children's emotional regulation and social cognition, as they learn to manage their emotions and consider the feelings of others.

Another key benefit of group play is that it encourages the development of leadership and decision-making skills. In group play, children often take on different roles, such as leader, follower, or mediator, depending on the dynamics of the group. These roles provide opportunities for children to practice making decisions, guiding others, and resolving conflicts, all of which contribute to the development of executive function and social competence.

While social interactions provide many cognitive benefits, some children face challenges in socialization during early childhood. These challenges can stem from a variety of factors, including developmental delays, behavioral issues, shyness, or environmental factors such as limited exposure to peers. Addressing these challenges is crucial for ensuring that all children have the opportunity to benefit from the cognitive growth that comes from social interaction.

For children who struggle with socialization, it is important to provide structured opportunities for social interaction in a supportive and low-pressure environment. For example, play-dates with one or two familiar peers may be less overwhelming than large group settings, allowing the child to practice social skills in a more manageable context. Additionally, adults can help facilitate social interactions by modeling appropriate behavior, encouraging turn-taking, and guiding children through conflict resolution.

For children with developmental delays or behavioral challenges, early intervention programs that focus on social skills development can be highly beneficial. These programs often include structured play activities that teach children how to interact with peers, manage their emotions, and solve problems in a social context. For example, a social skills group might focus on teaching children how to initiate conversations, interpret social cues, and respond appropriately to different social situations. These programs provide children with the tools they need to navigate social interactions more effectively, which in turn supports their cognitive development.

In cases where a child's socialization challenges are related to shyness or social anxiety, it is important for parents and caregivers to provide reassurance and support while gradually exposing the child to new social situations. Encouraging participation in activities that align with the child's interests—such as art classes, sports, or music lessons—can help build their confidence and provide opportunities for positive social interactions. Over time, as the child becomes more comfortable with socializing, they will begin to develop the cognitive and social skills that are fostered through peer interaction.

In conclusion, social interactions are a powerful driver of cognitive development in early childhood. Through engagement with peers, siblings, and adults, children develop problem-solving skills, executive function, and social cognition, all of which are essential for intellectual growth. Group play, in particular, provides a rich context for practicing these skills, as it requires children to navigate rules, share ideas, cooperate with others, and resolve conflicts. These experiences strengthen their ability to plan, focus, regulate their emotions, and adapt to changing situations. Social interactions offer countless opportunities for children to expand their thinking, learn from one another, and apply cognitive skills in real-world contexts.

For children who face challenges in socialization, it is crucial to offer support and create environments where they can practice and develop these skills. Structured and guided opportunities, such as small group activities, social skills programs, and low-pressure play-dates, can help children overcome barriers to social engagement and enable them to benefit from the cognitive growth that comes with interacting with peers and siblings. In the long run, addressing socialization challenges early on ensures that all children, regardless of their individual difficulties, have the opportunity to thrive cognitively and socially.

Parents, caregivers, and educators play a vital role in fostering these social experiences, providing guidance, support, and encouragement as children learn to navigate complex social dynamics. By promoting positive peer interactions, encouraging collaborative play, and creating opportunities for group activities, adults can help children develop essential cognitive skills that will serve them well in school and beyond. Social interactions not only contribute to intellectual growth but also build the foundation for emotional intelligence, empathy, and strong interpersonal relationships, which are just as important for a child's overall development.

In the end, socialization in early childhood is not merely about learning how to get along with others. It is about developing the cognitive tools necessary for critical thinking, problem-solving, and adaptability. Whether through play, cooperative learning, or sibling interactions, these social experiences shape a child's intellectual abilities and lay the groundwork for success in both academic and social spheres.

The Effects of Screen Time and Technology

The rapid integration of technology into daily life has significantly altered the way children learn, play, and interact with the world around them. In recent years, screen time has become a topic of growing concern, especially as children are introduced to digital devices such as smartphones, tablets, computers, and televisions at increasingly younger ages. With these changes, questions have emerged about the effects of screen time on cognitive development, the potential benefits of using technology for learning, and the importance of setting healthy boundaries for screen use. In this chapter, we will explore the current research on screen time and cognitive development, the effective use of technology to enhance learning, strategies for managing screen use, and the role of parental guidance in supporting healthy technology habits.

Over the past decade, a substantial body of research has emerged examining the effects of screen time on children's cognitive development. While technology and digital media can offer opportunities for learning and creativity, excessive or inappropriate use of screens has been linked to potential negative impacts on cognitive and behavioral development. Understanding the nuances of this research is essential for parents, educators, and caregivers as they navigate the complexities of raising children in a digital age.

One of the key concerns related to screen time is its impact on attention and executive function. Several studies have suggested that excessive screen use, particularly the use of fast-paced, highly stimulating media, may impair a child's ability to focus, regulate their emotions, and engage in sustained attention. This is particularly relevant when children are exposed to entertainment media, such as television shows or video games, that deliver constant stimuli in quick succession. Research has shown that children who consume large amounts of this type of content may struggle with attention regulation and impulse control, which can affect their academic performance and behavior in social settings.

Furthermore, the content and quality of screen time play a critical role in its impact on cognitive development. Passive consumption of entertainment media—such as watching television or YouTube videos—has been linked to delays in language development and lower levels of critical thinking skills. This is especially true for very young children (ages 0 to 3), whose developing brains are more vulnerable to the effects of excessive screen time. The American Academy of Pediatrics (AAP) recommends that children under the age of 18 months avoid screens altogether, except for video chatting, and that children between the ages of 2 and 5 have limited exposure, ideally no more than one hour of high-quality, educational content per day.

On the other hand, research has also shown that not all screen time is created equal, and certain types of digital content can have positive effects on cognitive development when used in moderation and under the right conditions. Educational apps, interactive games, and carefully curated media designed to promote learning can enhance cognitive skills such as problem-solving, memory, language development, and critical thinking. The key is to differentiate between passive and active screen time: passive screen time involves content where the child is a passive consumer, such as watching TV or non-interactive videos, whereas active screen time involves engaging with content that promotes participation, such as interactive games, coding programs, or educational apps that require thought and problem-solving.

Given the nuanced effects of screen time on cognitive development, it's essential for parents and educators to be intentional about how technology is integrated into children's daily lives. While there are legitimate concerns about the potential downsides of excessive screen time, technology also offers remarkable opportunities for enhancing learning when used appropriately. Educational apps, games, and digital tools have the potential to complement traditional learning methods, fostering creativity, problem-solving, and even collaboration in ways that were previously unavailable.

One of the most significant benefits of educational technology is its ability to provide personalized learning experiences. Interactive educational apps can adapt to a child's learning pace, offer immediate feedback, and present information in a variety of engaging formats. For example, apps that teach math or reading skills often use games and challenges to motivate children, helping them learn through play while simultaneously tracking their progress. Children who struggle with particular concepts can receive additional support through these apps, which offer targeted exercises designed to reinforce specific skills. These programs also allow children to work independently and build confidence in their abilities as they master new concepts.

Coding apps and games, such as Scratch or Mine craft Education Edition, have become popular tools for teaching children computational thinking, logic, and creativity. These platforms encourage children to build, problem-solve, and experiment with coding in a way that is accessible and fun. They promote both critical thinking and collaboration, as children can share their projects with peers and work together to create solutions to complex challenges. In this way, technology can enhance learning in ways that go beyond traditional methods, offering children new avenues for exploration and creativity.

Moreover, technology can enhance language development, particularly for bilingual children or those learning a second language. Interactive apps that focus on language acquisition provide opportunities for children to practice vocabulary, pronunciation, and comprehension in immersive environments. Some apps even incorporate real-time feedback through voice recognition, helping children correct their pronunciation and improve fluency in a language that might not be spoken frequently at home. This personalized, interactive approach to language learning has been shown to be effective in developing communication skills and expanding a child's vocabulary.

Additionally, digital tools can promote scientific inquiry and critical thinking by allowing children to experiment with virtual simulations. Apps and websites that offer science-related content, such as virtual labs or exploration tools, enable children to explore scientific concepts in a hands-on, interactive manner. These resources allow children to conduct experiments, observe phenomena, and test hypotheses in a virtual setting, all of which foster curiosity and deeper understanding of the world around them. In classrooms, technology-based tools like interactive whiteboards and tablets enable teachers to demonstrate complex concepts visually, making abstract ideas more accessible and engaging for students.

Despite the educational benefits of technology, it is crucial to set healthy boundaries around screen use to ensure that children develop a balanced relationship with technology. Screen time should not replace physical activity, face-to-face social interactions, or unstructured play, all of which are essential for healthy cognitive and emotional development. Research shows that children who spend excessive time on screens are at higher risk for physical health issues such as obesity and sleep disturbances, as well as emotional problems like anxiety and depression. To mitigate these risks, parents should establish clear limits on screen use and encourage a variety of activities that promote overall well-being.

One effective strategy for setting healthy boundaries is to create a structured routine that includes designated screen time as well as time for other activities, such as outdoor play, reading, family interactions, and creative play. For example, parents might designate one hour after school for educational apps or games, followed by outdoor playtime or family meals with no screens allowed. This structured approach helps children understand that screens are just one part of a balanced day and reinforces the importance of engaging in a variety of activities.

It is also important to set clear rules regarding when and where screens can be used. For instance, many experts recommend establishing screen-free zones in the home, such as the dining room or bedroom, to promote healthy habits. Keeping screens out of the bedroom can help prevent sleep disruptions, which are often caused by the blue light emitted from digital devices. Additionally, setting aside device-free family time, such as during meals or outings, allows for meaningful interactions and promotes family bonding without the distraction of screens.

In addition to managing the amount of screen time, parents should also be mindful of the content their children are consuming. Ensuring that children have access to high-quality, age-appropriate content is essential for making the most of screen time. Parents can use tools such as parental controls, app ratings, and reviews to evaluate the suitability of apps, games, and websites for their child's developmental level. Platforms like Common Sense Media provide valuable insights and recommendations on digital content, helping parents make informed choices about the media their children engage with.

The role of parental guidance in managing technology exposure cannot be overstated. Children learn how to use technology not only from the apps and programs they engage with but also from observing how their parents and caregivers use technology. Parental involvement is key to helping children develop healthy technology habits, and this begins with modeling responsible screen use. Parents who set clear boundaries for their own screen time, limit distractions during family interactions, and demonstrate the value of offline activities send a strong message to their children about the importance of balance.

Parents can also play an active role in co-viewing and co-playing with their children. Engaging with children during screen time provides an opportunity to discuss what they are learning, ask questions that deepen their understanding, and guide them toward making thoughtful choices about the content they consume. Co-viewing also allows parents to reinforce lessons from educational programs or games and help children make connections between what they see on screen and the real world. For example, after watching an educational video about animals, a parent might take their child to the zoo or read a related book to expand on the learning experience.

Open communication about technology is another essential aspect of parental guidance. As children grow older and begin to use technology more independently, it is important for parents to have ongoing conversations about responsible digital citizenship. This includes discussing topics such as online safety, appropriate behavior on social media, the importance of critical thinking when evaluating online information, and the risks of excessive screen time. By fostering an open dialogue, parents can help children develop the skills they need to navigate the digital world safely and responsibly.

In conclusion, screen time and technology have both positive and negative implications for cognitive development, depending on how they are used. While excessive and unregulated screen use can lead to issues such as attention difficulties, behavioral problems, and impaired social skills, technology can also be a powerful tool for learning when used thoughtfully and in moderation. Educational apps, interactive games, and digital tools offer opportunities for personalized learning, creativity, and problem-solving, making technology a valuable resource for cognitive development.

To ensure that children benefit from the advantages of technology while avoiding its pitfalls, it is essential for parents and caregivers to set healthy boundaries around screen use, provide access to high-quality content, and model responsible technology habits. Parental guidance plays a critical role in helping children develop a balanced relationship with technology, one that fosters both intellectual growth and emotional well-being.

Parents must not only set limits but also actively engage with their children in meaningful ways to ensure that technology use remains balanced, educational, and productive. This includes teaching children how to critically engage with content, encouraging them to ask questions, and guiding them toward content that promotes learning rather than passive consumption. The conversations around technology need to evolve as children grow, with parents playing a continuous role in shaping their child's understanding of digital responsibility, online safety, and healthy screen habits.

As children become more independent and screen time inevitably increases— whether for educational purposes or leisure—parental involvement becomes even more important. This is where teaching digital literacy becomes critical. Digital literacy extends beyond knowing how to operate devices or apps. It involves understanding the quality and credibility of content, recognizing potential biases in the media, and being aware of the risks associated with online interactions, such as exposure to inappropriate content or cyberbully. Educating children about the importance of privacy, not sharing personal information online, and recognizing potential dangers in the digital world are all essential aspects of digital literacy that can prevent harm and ensure a safe online experience.

One way parents can support digital literacy is by providing guided experiences with technology. For example, when a child uses a search engine for schoolwork, parents can guide them on how to distinguish reliable sources from unreliable ones. In addition, parents can discuss with their children the importance of thinking critically about the information they come across online. By fostering these skills early on, parents help children become more discerning users of technology who can navigate the digital world confidently and responsibly.

In terms of managing screen time, it is important for parents to understand the concept of balance rather than relying solely on time-based restrictions. Not all screen time is equal, and focusing on the quality of time spent on screens is more beneficial than adhering to strict limits. Educational apps, creative software, and interactive games that stimulate thinking and creativity are far more beneficial to a child's cognitive development than passively watching entertainment content for the same amount of time. A child who spends an hour learning to code or creating digital artwork is engaging in cognitively enriching activities, whereas an hour spent watching non-educational videos may have limited benefits.

To foster a balanced approach to technology, it can be helpful for families to adopt a "media diet" approach, similar to a balanced food diet. This media diet should include a variety of activities, such as physical play, reading, social interactions, and creative projects, alongside screen time. By framing technology as one part of a child's broader learning and development experience, parents can help their children appreciate the benefits of moderation and variety in their daily lives. Integrating technology use with non-screen activities is a practical way to achieve balance. For instance, if a child is interested in a particular topic they encountered through an app or game, parents can encourage them to explore that topic further through books, outdoor activities, or hands-on projects that connect the digital experience with the real world.

Moreover, one of the most important aspects of setting healthy boundaries is ensuring that screen time does not interfere with sleep, physical activity, or face-to-face interactions. Research consistently shows that excessive screen use—particularly before bedtime—can disrupt sleep patterns, leading to fatigue and concentration difficulties the next day. This is because the blue light emitted from screens can interfere with the body's production of melanin, a hormone that regulates sleep. To avoid sleep disruptions, it is recommended that screens be turned off at least one hour before bedtime, and that children's bedrooms remain screen-free zones. In this way, children can establish healthy sleep routines that support overall cognitive and emotional well-being.

Ensuring that technology use is balanced with physical activity is also essential for a child's development. Physical movement is crucial for brain health, as it improves blood flow to the brain, enhances memory, and supports cognitive functioning. Encouraging children to engage in active play, whether indoors or outdoors, helps them build important motor skills and strengthens their cognitive abilities. Parents can set a positive example by prioritizing physical activity as part of the family's daily routine and offering fun, engaging ways for children to stay active, such as playing sports, hiking, or biking.

Finally, face-to-face social interactions should always take precedence over screen-based communication. While digital platforms offer ways to stay connected with friends and family, they cannot replace the richness of in-person interactions, which are essential for developing emotional intelligence, empathy, and social skills. Engaging in real-life conversations, collaborating with peers, and participating in group activities help children learn how to navigate social dynamics, understand body language, and express their emotions effectively. By promoting screen-free time during family meals, outings, and social events, parents can create opportunities for meaningful interactions that strengthen their child's social and emotional development.

Parental involvement in managing technology exposure goes beyond setting rules and enforcing limits; it involves fostering a healthy relationship with technology that encourages critical thinking, creativity, and balance. This means encouraging children to use technology as a tool for learning and self-expression rather than as a passive form of entertainment or distraction. When technology is used thoughtfully and in moderation, it has the potential to enhance a child's cognitive development, support academic success, and foster a lifelong love of learning.

In addition to fostering healthy habits at home, parents should also be mindful of how schools are integrating technology into the learning environment. Many schools have adopted one-to-one technology initiatives, where each student is provided with a personal device, such as a tablet or laptop, to enhance learning. While these initiatives can offer opportunities for personalized learning and digital engagement, they also require careful oversight to ensure that technology is being used effectively and responsibly. Parents can support their child's use of educational technology by staying informed about the school's technology policies, discussing the content being covered in class, and encouraging their child to reflect on how technology is enhancing their learning experience.

Ultimately, the goal is to help children develop a balanced and healthy relationship with technology that supports their cognitive, social, and emotional development. As digital devices become increasingly integrated into daily life, teaching children how to use these tools responsibly and intentionally is essential for their overall well-being. By guiding children through the complexities of the digital world, setting clear boundaries, and promoting a variety of enriching activities, parents can help their children thrive in an increasingly technology-driven society.

In conclusion, the effects of screen time and technology on cognitive development are multifaceted, requiring a nuanced approach from parents, educators, and caregivers. While excessive screen time can lead to issues such as attention difficulties, behavioral problems, and impaired social skills, technology also has the potential to be a powerful tool for learning when used thoughtfully and in moderation. Educational apps, interactive games, and digital tools can foster creativity, problem-solving, and personalized learning experiences that support cognitive growth.

To ensure that technology is used in a way that enhances learning and development, it is essential to set healthy boundaries around screen use, provide access to high-quality educational content, and maintain a balanced approach to daily activities. Parents play a pivotal role in guiding their children's technology use, modeling responsible behavior, and fostering open communication about the benefits and risks of the digital world. By doing so, they can help their children develop the skills they need to navigate technology responsibly, while also supporting their cognitive and emotional well-being. Through mindful use of technology and a focus on balance, parents can create an environment where children can benefit from the advantages of the digital age while avoiding its potential pitfalls.

Encouraging Problem-Solving and Critical Thinking Skills

Encouraging problem-solving and critical thinking skills in children is one of the most effective ways to nurture cognitive growth. These skills are essential not only for academic success but also for navigating life's challenges, making informed decisions, and developing a mindset geared towards creativity and innovation. Problem-solving and critical thinking help children analyze situations, think logically, and explore multiple solutions to a given problem. To foster these abilities, parents and educators can implement strategies that encourage curiosity, decision-making, and exploration, creating an environment where children feel empowered to think independently and engage with the world around them.

Fostering curiosity and a sense of wonder is the foundation of developing critical thinking and problem-solving skills in children. Curiosity drives children to explore, ask questions, and seek out knowledge, which are all essential components of cognitive growth. By nurturing a child's natural curiosity, parents and educators can inspire a lifelong love of learning and an openness to new ideas.

One of the most effective ways to encourage curiosity is to create an environment where questioning is valued and welcomed. Children are naturally inquisitive, often asking "why" about the world around them. Instead of providing direct answers to every question, adults can foster deeper thinking by responding with questions of their own, such as, "What do you think?" or "How could we find out?" These open-ended questions encourage children to reflect on their own understanding, form hypotheses, and explore possible solutions.

In addition, adults can model curiosity by expressing their own interest in learning and discovery. For example, when a parent or teacher encounters a new concept or situation, they can express curiosity aloud, saying, "I wonder why this happens," or "Let's see if we can figure this out together." By demonstrating a curiosity-driven approach to learning, adults show children that it is okay not to have all the answers and that exploration and investigation are valuable parts of the learning process.

Encouraging children to engage in activities that naturally inspire curiosity is another effective strategy. For instance, providing opportunities for hands-on exploration, such as nature walks, science experiments, or building projects, can spark children's interest in learning how things work. When children are actively involved in discovering answers for themselves, they are more likely to develop critical thinking and problem-solving skills as they learn to observe, experiment, and draw conclusions.

Another technique for fostering curiosity is to introduce children to a wide variety of experiences and perspectives. Exposure to different cultures, ideas, and fields of knowledge can broaden their understanding of the world and inspire them to ask questions about subjects they may not have previously considered. This can be accomplished through activities such as reading books on diverse topics, visiting museums, engaging in cultural experiences, or learning about science, history, and the arts in a way that captures their imagination.

Teaching children how to make decisions and solve problems is a key component of building cognitive resilience and critical thinking. Decision-making and problem-solving require children to evaluate information, weigh options, and consider potential outcomes before arriving at a solution. These skills can be developed through intentional practices that guide children in thinking through problems rather than solving them for them.

One of the most important steps in teaching decision-making is to involve children in everyday choices from a young age. Even simple decisions, such as choosing what to wear, selecting a snack, or picking an activity, help children practice evaluating options and making choices based on their preferences or needs. As children grow older, the decisions can become more complex, involving factors such as time management, balancing responsibilities, or considering the consequences of their actions.

When guiding children through decision-making, it is helpful to break the process down into manageable steps. For example, parents and educators can teach children to:
1. Identify the problem or decision that needs to be made.
2. Gather information or consider the available options.
3. Evaluate the pros and cons of each option.
4. Choose a course of action based on their evaluation.
5. Reflect on the outcome to learn from the experience.

This structured approach provides a framework that children can apply in different contexts, helping them develop confidence in their ability to make decisions independently. It is important to allow children to experience the consequences of their decisions—both positive and negative—so that they learn from their mistakes and successes. This builds resilience and helps children understand that problem-solving is a process that often involves trial and error.

Problem-solving can also be encouraged through collaborative activities that require children to work together to find solutions. Group projects, games, or discussions that involve multiple perspectives can help children learn how to approach problems creatively, listen to others' ideas, and consider alternative solutions. For example, working together to build a structure, solve a puzzle, or create a story encourages children to negotiate roles, share ideas, and adapt their thinking based on input from others. These experiences enhance their ability to think critically and collaborate effectively with peers.

One of the most engaging and effective ways to enhance thinking skills in children is through puzzles, games, and activities that challenge their cognitive abilities. These activities provide opportunities for children to practice problem-solving, logical reasoning, spatial awareness, and critical thinking in a fun and interactive way.

Puzzles, such as jigsaw puzzles, crossword puzzles, or Sudoku, require children to use reasoning, pattern recognition, and attention to detail. As they work to solve these puzzles, children must think critically about how the pieces fit together or how to approach a problem from different angles. Puzzles also encourage perseverance and patience, as children may need to try multiple approaches before finding the correct solution.

Board games that involve strategy, such as chess, checkers, or Risk, are another excellent way to develop critical thinking skills. These games require players to plan ahead, anticipate their opponent's moves, and adapt their strategy based on changing circumstances. By playing these games, children learn to think strategically, make decisions based on available information, and adjust their approach when faced with new challenges.

Interactive digital games and apps that promote problem-solving and logic can also be valuable tools for enhancing thinking skills. Games that involve coding, building, or problem-solving—such as Mine craft, Scratch, or logic puzzles—allow children to experiment with different solutions, build structures, and develop their computational thinking skills. Many educational apps offer challenges that adapt to the child's skill level, providing increasing levels of complexity that help strengthen critical thinking and problem-solving abilities over time.

Activities that involve building and construction, such as using LEGO blocks, K'nex, or other building sets, encourage spatial reasoning, engineering skills, and creativity. Children must think critically about how to design and construct structures, solve problems related to stability and balance, and use their imagination to create something new. These hands-on activities provide a tangible way for children to apply problem-solving strategies and explore different possibilities.

Additionally, activities that promote creative thinking, such as art projects, storytelling, or role-playing, encourage children to think outside the box and explore alternative solutions to problems. For example, in art, children might be faced with the challenge of figuring out how to create a particular effect using different materials or techniques. In storytelling or role-playing, children must develop narratives, create characters, and solve conflicts within the story, all of which require them to use their imagination and critical thinking skills.

Encouraging exploration and independent learning is essential for fostering problem-solving and critical thinking. Children who are given the freedom to explore their interests, experiment with new ideas, and engage in self-directed learning are more likely to develop a growth mindset and a sense of curiosity about the world. Independent learning allows children to take ownership of their education, pursue topics that interest them, and apply their problem-solving skills in real-world contexts.

One way to encourage independent learning is by creating an environment where children have access to a variety of resources that support exploration. This might include books, art supplies, building materials, science kits, or technology tools that allow children to investigate different subjects on their own. By providing children with the tools they need to explore their interests, parents and educators can create a space where independent learning is both encouraged and celebrated.

Allowing children to pursue projects that interest them is another effective way to foster independent learning. For example, if a child is interested in animals, they might research different species, create a model habitat, or write a report about their favorite animal. These types of projects encourage children to apply their problem-solving and critical thinking skills as they gather information, organize their findings, and present their ideas.

Exploration can also be encouraged through outdoor play and nature-based activities. Time spent in nature provides endless opportunities for inquiry and investigation, whether through observing wildlife, conducting simple experiments, or exploring natural environments. Outdoor exploration fosters curiosity, creativity, and problem-solving as children engage with the world around them and learn to adapt to new challenges.

Finally, parents and educators can promote independent learning by encouraging children to set goals and reflect on their progress. By helping children identify areas of interest, set achievable goals, and evaluate their successes and challenges, adults can foster a sense of ownership over the learning process. This not only builds confidence but also encourages children to take an active role in their own education, applying problem-solving and critical thinking skills to achieve their objectives.

In conclusion, fostering problem-solving and critical thinking skills in children requires intentional strategies that encourage curiosity, decision-making, and exploration. By creating an environment where questioning is valued, children are given opportunities to engage in activities that challenge their thinking, and they are encouraged to pursue independent learning, parents and educators can help children develop the cognitive skills they need to succeed in school and in life. Through puzzles, games, hands-on activities, and real-world experiences, children can practice problem-solving in a variety of contexts, building the critical thinking abilities that will serve them well throughout their lives.

As children continue to engage with the world around them, the skills they develop through problem-solving and critical thinking extend beyond the classroom and into everyday life. These abilities equip them to navigate complex social situations, handle challenges with resilience, and approach new experiences with confidence. The goal is not just to help children excel academically, but to empower them with the tools they need to be independent thinkers, capable of making informed decisions and solving problems creatively in a variety of contexts.

One of the key benefits of fostering these skills is that it prepares children to handle uncertainty and ambiguity. In life, not all problems have clear solutions, and there are often multiple ways to approach a challenge. By encouraging children to explore different possibilities and think critically about their options, parents and educators can help them become comfortable with ambiguity and uncertainty. This mindset is essential for adapting to change, as it allows children to remain flexible and open to new ideas rather than becoming rigid in their thinking.

Another important aspect of developing problem-solving and critical thinking skills is that it promotes resilience. When children are given the freedom to experiment, make mistakes, and learn from their experiences, they develop a growth mindset—a belief that intelligence and abilities can be developed through effort and persistence. This mindset helps children view challenges as opportunities for growth rather than obstacles to be avoided. When they encounter a difficult task, they are more likely to persevere, try different strategies, and learn from their mistakes rather than giving up. Over time, this resilience not only enhances their problem-solving abilities but also builds their confidence in tackling new challenges.

In addition, encouraging exploration and independent learning helps children develop a sense of autonomy and self-motivation. When children are given the opportunity to pursue their interests, make decisions, and solve problems on their own, they take ownership of their learning and become more intrinsically motivated to explore new ideas. This intrinsic motivation is a key factor in fostering a love of learning that extends beyond the classroom. Children who are self-motivated are more likely to continue seeking out new knowledge and experiences throughout their lives, which is essential for both personal and intellectual growth.

One of the most powerful ways to nurture this sense of autonomy is by allowing children to take risks in their learning. Risk-taking, in this context, doesn't mean engaging in unsafe behaviors, but rather being willing to try new things, experiment with different approaches, and step outside of one's comfort zone. When children are encouraged to take intellectual risks—whether by attempting a challenging puzzle, trying a new activity, or presenting an original idea—they learn to embrace uncertainty and see failure as a natural part of the learning process. This helps them build confidence in their ability to solve problems and think critically, even when the outcome is uncertain.

Parents and educators play a critical role in creating a safe environment for risk-taking by offering support, encouragement, and guidance without being overly controlling. When children feel that they have the freedom to make mistakes without fear of judgment or punishment, they are more likely to take the kinds of risks that lead to meaningful learning and growth. For example, when a child is struggling with a math problem, instead of providing the solution right away, an adult might offer a suggestion or ask a guiding question that encourages the child to think through the problem on their own. This approach helps children develop confidence in their own problem-solving abilities and fosters a sense of ownership over their learning.

Furthermore, collaboration and peer learning are valuable components of developing critical thinking and problem-solving skills. Working with others provides children with opportunities to encounter different perspectives, share ideas, and learn from one another. When children collaborate on projects, they must communicate effectively, negotiate roles, and solve problems together, all of which enhance their cognitive flexibility and social skills. Group activities, such as team-based games, cooperative building projects, or group discussions, provide a rich context for children to practice these skills in a dynamic and interactive environment.

Encouraging peer learning also helps children develop empathy and the ability to consider others' viewpoints, both of which are essential for effective problem-solving. When children work together, they learn to listen to each other's ideas, incorporate feedback, and develop solutions that take into account the needs and perspectives of the group. These experiences not only enhance their cognitive abilities but also promote social-emotional growth, as they learn to navigate the complexities of working in a team and resolving conflicts.

In addition to peer learning, mentorship can be a valuable tool for fostering problem-solving and critical thinking skills. A mentor—whether a parent, teacher, or older peer—can provide guidance, model effective thinking strategies, and offer feedback that helps the child develop their cognitive abilities. Mentors can help children approach problems in a structured way, encourage them to think critically about their options, and support them in finding solutions that work for them. For example, a teacher might mentor a student by helping them develop a study plan for a challenging subject, breaking the problem down into manageable steps, and offering support and feedback along the way. This type of guidance helps children build the skills and confidence they need to tackle problems independently.

Technology can also be a valuable tool for nurturing problem-solving and critical thinking, provided it is used thoughtfully and in moderation. Educational apps, online games, and digital tools can provide children with interactive, engaging experiences that challenge their thinking and encourage them to solve problems in creative ways. For example, coding programs like Scratch allow children to experiment with creating their own games and animations, teaching them logic, sequencing, and computational thinking in a fun and accessible way. Similarly, digital puzzles and strategy games can help children develop their problem-solving abilities by presenting them with complex challenges that require planning, strategy, and adaptability.

However, it is important for parents and educators to ensure that technology is used as a tool for learning rather than a replacement for hands-on experiences. While digital tools can offer valuable learning opportunities, they should be balanced with real-world exploration, physical play, and face-to-face interactions. Children need opportunities to engage in creative play, build with their hands, and interact with the natural world to develop their full range of cognitive and problem-solving abilities. By providing a balanced approach to technology use, adults can help children harness the benefits of digital learning while ensuring that they continue to engage with the world around them in meaningful and enriching ways.

Ultimately, fostering problem-solving and critical thinking skills in children is about creating a supportive environment where exploration, curiosity, and intellectual risk-taking are encouraged. By providing opportunities for hands-on learning, offering guidance and mentorship, and encouraging children to engage in activities that challenge their thinking, parents and educators can help children develop the cognitive tools they need to succeed both in school and in life. These skills—critical thinking, problem-solving, decision-making, and resilience—are essential for navigating the complexities of the modern world and for fostering a mindset that embraces lifelong learning and growth.

In summary, the development of problem-solving and critical thinking skills is a dynamic and multifaceted process that requires intentional effort from parents, educators, and the children themselves. By fostering curiosity, providing opportunities for decision-making, encouraging independent exploration, and incorporating puzzles, games, and collaborative activities into daily learning, adults can create an environment where children are empowered to think critically and solve problems creatively. This approach not only enhances cognitive development but also instills in children the confidence and resilience they need to tackle challenges and embrace new experiences with enthusiasm and curiosity.

Developing Attention, Focus, and Memory

The development of attention, focus, and memory is foundational for a child's cognitive growth. These skills are integral to learning, problem-solving, and emotional regulation. From infancy through early childhood, children gradually develop the ability to concentrate for longer periods, focus on tasks, and retain information. Understanding how these abilities evolve and the strategies that can enhance them is crucial for parents, educators, and caregivers in nurturing a child's intellectual capabilities.

Attention span is the ability to focus on a particular task or object for a period of time, and its development begins in infancy and continues through childhood. Early in life, infants have very short attention spans, often shifting their focus quickly from one object to another as they explore their environment. At this stage, attention is primarily driven by sensory experiences, such as sounds, sights, and textures, which stimulate curiosity and engagement. However, as children grow, they begin to develop the cognitive control necessary to maintain their focus on a single task or activity for longer periods.

The growth of attention span in young children is influenced by both biological and environmental factors. Neurological development, particularly the maturation of the prefrontal cortex, plays a significant role in a child's ability to focus and regulate their attention. This part of the brain is responsible for executive functions, which include planning, decision-making, and inhibitory control—the ability to block out distractions and sustain focus on a task. As the prefrontal cortex develops, children gain greater control over their attention and can concentrate on more complex activities.

Environmental factors, such as the presence of supportive and stimulating learning environments, also impact the development of attention. Children who are exposed to rich, engaging activities that challenge their thinking and captivate their interest are more likely to develop longer attention spans. On the other hand, environments with constant distractions or over stimulation—such as excessive screen time or chaotic surroundings—can hinder the development of sustained focus. It is essential for parents and caregivers to create a balanced environment that promotes both exploration and concentration, allowing children to naturally extend their attention span as they engage with the world around them.

In terms of developmental milestones, attention span gradually increases as children grow. Toddlers may only be able to focus on a task for a few minutes at a time, while preschoolers can typically concentrate for longer periods, especially if the activity is of interest to them. By the time children enter school, their ability to sustain attention for structured activities, such as listening to a story or completing a puzzle, is significantly enhanced. However, each child develops at their own pace, and attention spans can vary widely based on individual temperament, interests, and experiences.

Building focus in young children requires intentional strategies that align with their developmental stage. Since young children are naturally curious and easily distracted, it is important to introduce activities that capture their interest and gradually challenge their ability to concentrate. One effective strategy is to start with short, engaging tasks and gradually increase their complexity and duration as the child's attention span grows. For instance, parents and educators can begin with simple activities, such as stacking blocks or matching colors, and slowly introduce more intricate puzzles or games that require sustained concentration.

Structured routines are another powerful tool for building focus in young children. Routines provide a sense of predictability and structure, helping children understand what is expected of them and when. When children know that certain times are designated for specific activities—such as playtime, reading, or quiet time—they are more likely to focus on the task at hand without becoming easily distracted. For example, a daily routine that includes a set time for reading or art projects encourages children to engage in those activities with more focus, as they become accustomed to the rhythm of the day.

Minimizing distractions is also critical for promoting focus. In a world filled with digital devices, loud noises, and constant stimuli, children can find it challenging to concentrate on a single task. Creating a calm and distraction-free environment helps children focus more effectively. This can be achieved by turning off the television or limiting access to electronic devices during specific activities, such as mealtime or study time. Additionally, providing a designated space for quiet activities—such as a reading nook or a study area—can help children associate that space with focus and concentration.

Parents and educators can further support focus by offering positive rein-forcement and encouragement when children successfully complete tasks or demonstrate sustained attention. Praise for effort, rather than just results, reinforces the importance of persistence and helps children develop confidence in their ability to focus. For example, acknowledging a child's hard work in completing a puzzle or finishing a drawing encourages them to continue engaging in tasks that require concentration.

Another strategy for building focus is through physical movement and breaks. Children, especially young ones, need opportunities to move their bodies and release energy, as this can actually improve their ability to concentrate. Incorporating short, active breaks between periods of focused activity can help reset a child's attention and make it easier for them to return to the task at hand. For instance, after spending time on a quiet activity like reading, allowing children to run, jump, or play for a few minutes helps them expend energy and refocus when it's time to return to a more structured task.

Memory is another essential component of cognitive development, and children's ability to remember information improves significantly during the early years. Memory-building games and activities are a fun and effective way to enhance a child's recall, working memory, and long-term memory skills. These activities not only support cognitive growth but also lay the foundation for academic success, as memory plays a crucial role in learning new concepts and retaining information.

Memory games, such as matching card games or "Simon Says," require children to remember patterns, sequences, or instructions, which helps strengthen their working memory. These games can be easily adapted to different ages and skill levels, making them accessible for toddlers and older children alike. For example, a simple matching game with picture cards can be used to improve visual memory, while a game like "Simon Says" encourages children to remember and follow multiple-step instructions, enhancing their auditory memory and attention to detail.

Repetition is a key factor in building memory, and incorporating repetition into daily activities can help reinforce memory skills. For instance, parents can ask children to recall what they did earlier in the day or what they learned at school. Asking open-ended questions, such as "What was your favorite part of the story?" or "Can you remember what happened next?" encourages children to practice recalling information. This type of informal recall activity strengthens both short-term and long-term memory by encouraging children to actively retrieve information from their memory banks.

Storytelling is another powerful tool for memory building. When children are encouraged to tell their own stories or retell a story they have heard, they are practicing sequencing, recall, and organization of information. This not only enhances memory but also promotes language development and creative thinking. Storytelling activities can be as simple as asking a child to describe their day in order or retelling a favorite bedtime story, with the added challenge of remembering key details or events.

Songs and rhymes are also effective memory-building tools. Many traditional children's songs and nursery rhymes are designed with repetition and rhythm, which make them easier for children to remember. Singing songs together or playing memory-based musical games helps children practice auditory memory and recall patterns, which are important for learning language and early literacy skills.

In addition to games and activities, visual aids such as charts, picture sequences, and memory maps can help children build memory by associating information with images. For example, creating a picture schedule for the day's activities helps children remember the sequence of events and builds their ability to recall routines. Visual cues, such as storyboards or drawings, can also help children remember the order of events in a story or process, making it easier for them to recall details when asked.

However, some children may experience challenges in developing attention and focus, which can be related to underlying conditions such as attention deficit hyperactivity disorder (ADHD) or other attention-related disorders. Managing attention disorders in early childhood requires a compassionate, structured, and supportive approach that helps children build focus while accommodating their unique needs.

For children with ADHD or similar disorders, maintaining focus on tasks can be especially difficult, as they may become easily distracted or impulsive. These children often struggle with sustaining attention, completing tasks, and regulating their behavior, which can impact their learning and social interactions. Early intervention and support are critical for helping children with attention disorders develop strategies to manage their symptoms and succeed in school and life.

One effective approach for managing attention disorders is to break tasks into smaller, more manageable steps. Children with attention difficulties may feel overwhelmed by large tasks, which can lead to frustration and disengagement. By breaking tasks into smaller chunks and providing clear, simple instructions, parents and educators can help children focus on one step at a time. For example, rather than asking a child to clean their entire room at once, parents can guide them to start by picking up their toys, then move on to another part of the task. This method not only makes the task feel more achievable but also helps children practice focusing on one task before moving on to the next.

Structured routines are also highly beneficial for children with attention disorders. Predictable routines help children know what to expect and reduce the anxiety or impulsivity that can arise from sudden transitions or unexpected changes. Having consistent routines for activities such as mealtimes, playtime, and bedtime provides a sense of stability and helps children develop the ability to focus during specific periods of the day. For children with ADHD, visual schedules or checklists can be particularly helpful in organizing their tasks and maintaining focus.

In addition to routines, incorporating movement and sensory breaks into the day is essential for children with attention disorders. These children often have excess energy or sensory needs that make it difficult for them to sit still or concentrate for extended periods. Short breaks for physical activity, such as jumping, stretching, or running, help them release pent-up energy and reset their attention. Sensory activities, such as playing with fidget toys, using weighted blankets, or engaging in deep-pressure touch, can also help calm their bodies and improve focus.

Positive reinforcement and encouragement are crucial for children with attention disorders. Recognizing and rewarding their efforts to focus, even if the task isn't completed perfectly, reinforces the idea that concentration and persistence are valuable. Rather than focusing on the child's struggles with attention, it is essential to celebrate small successes and provide praise when they demonstrate focus or complete a task, no matter how minor. Positive reinforcement helps build self-esteem and encourages the child to keep trying, fostering a growth mindset where they believe their attention skills can improve with effort.

Parents and educators should also be mindful of setting realistic expectations for children with attention disorders. It is important to recognize that these children may need more time or support to complete tasks that others might find easy. Being patient and adjusting the demands placed on the child to match their attention capacity helps prevent feelings of frustration or failure. Instead of expecting a child with ADHD to sit still and focus for the same length of time as their peers, caregivers can gradually increase the time spent on focused activities, giving the child opportunities to build up their attention span at their own pace.

In some cases, therapeutic interventions such as behavioral therapy or occupational therapy can be highly beneficial for children with attention disorders. Behavioral therapy often focuses on helping children develop strategies for managing impulsivity, regulating their emotions, and improving focus. Therapists work with children to develop coping mechanisms and routines that make it easier for them to succeed in daily tasks and social interactions. Occupational therapy can also support children with sensory processing challenges that may contribute to difficulties with attention, offering tools and activities to improve their ability to concentrate in different environments.

Another essential aspect of managing attention disorders is communication between parents, educators, and healthcare professionals. A team-based approach ensures that everyone involved in the child's care is on the same page and that strategies used at home and in school are consistent. Regular check-ins with teachers, therapists, or pediatricians help monitor the child's progress and make adjustments to their support plan as needed. This collaborative effort maximizes the child's ability to build focus, attention, and memory skills in a supportive and structured manner.

Technology can also be leveraged as a tool for managing attention disorders and improving focus. Several apps and digital tools are designed to help children with ADHD manage their time, stay organized, and focus on tasks. For example, apps that use timers or visual schedules can help children stay on track with their daily routines, while reward-based apps can motivate them to complete tasks and focus for specific intervals. While technology should be used in moderation and balanced with non-digital activities, it can provide additional structure and support for children with attention challenges.

Additionally, it is essential to remember that each child is unique, and what works for one child may not work for another. Some children respond well to structured environments and routines, while others may need more flexibility and opportunities for movement. Tailoring strategies to the individual child's needs, temperament, and strengths is critical to helping them develop their attention, focus, and memory skills.

Developing attention, focus, and memory in children is a dynamic and ongoing process that requires a combination of environmental support, intentional strategies, and individual attention to each child's needs. Through games, structured activities, and positive reinforcement, parents and educators can help children build the cognitive skills necessary for learning and everyday life. For children with attention disorders, managing focus requires patience, understanding, and a tailored approach that accommodates their specific challenges while encouraging growth.

Ultimately, fostering these abilities in early childhood lays the foundation for lifelong success. As children learn to manage their attention and improve their focus and memory, they become more equipped to handle the complexities of academic learning, social interactions, and problem-solving.

Whether through memory-building games, carefully structured routines, or individualized support for attention disorders, nurturing these skills will help children develop the cognitive resilience they need to thrive in an increasingly demanding world.

Fostering Creativity and Imagination

Creativity and imagination are not only vital components of artistic expression but also play crucial roles in cognitive growth and overall development. For children, creativity fuels problem-solving, critical thinking, and the ability to think abstractly. It provides a foundation for cognitive flexibility, allowing young minds to adapt to new information, develop innovative ideas, and understand the world in complex, nuanced ways. Fostering creativity is essential for nurturing a child's cognitive, emotional, and social development, and it supports the skills they need to thrive in both academic and personal pursuits. Encouraging creative thinking and expression can be achieved through a variety of strategies and activities that allow children to explore their imagination, experiment with new ideas, and engage in artistic, musical, and dramatic play.

The connection between creativity and cognitive growth is profound. Creativity requires children to think beyond the obvious, make connections between seemingly unrelated ideas, and explore multiple solutions to problems. This type of thinking strengthens cognitive flexibility, which is the ability to shift between different concepts, adapt to new situations, and approach challenges from different perspectives. Cognitive flexibility is essential for problem-solving, critical thinking, and the ability to learn new information.

When children engage in creative activities, such as drawing, storytelling, or building with blocks, they are practicing the skills that underlie cognitive growth. For example, when a child draws a picture, they are not only expressing their artistic vision but also making decisions about color, shape, and composition. They are using their imagination to bring an idea to life, which requires them to think abstractly and visualize possibilities. Similarly, when children engage in pretend play, they are creating imaginary scenarios that involve complex narratives, roles, and rules. This type of play encourages children to think critically about how to solve problems within the context of their imaginative world, which in turn strengthens their cognitive abilities.

Creativity also enhances memory and attention by requiring children to focus on the task at hand and remember the details of their creative process. For instance, when children create a story or a piece of artwork, they must remember the sequence of events or the elements they have already included in their composition. This strengthens their working memory and helps them develop the ability to organize and structure information in meaningful ways.

Moreover, creativity supports emotional regulation and self-expression. Children often use creative outlets, such as drawing, music, or play, to express their feelings and work through complex emotions. This process allows them to develop emotional intelligence, which is the ability to understand and manage their own emotions and respond to the emotions of others. Emotional intelligence is closely linked to cognitive growth, as it supports social interactions, problem-solving, and decision-making.

Encouraging creative thinking and expression in children begins with creating an environment that values and nurtures creativity. One of the most important aspects of fostering creativity is providing children with the freedom to explore their ideas without fear of failure or judgment. Creativity thrives in an environment where children feel safe to take risks, make mistakes, and experiment with new concepts. Adults can support this by offering positive reinforcement for effort rather than focusing solely on the outcome of a creative project. For example, instead of praising a child only for the finished product, such as a drawing or a sculpture, parents and educators can praise the child's creativity, imagination, and willingness to try something new.

Open-ended questions are another powerful tool for encouraging creative thinking. Asking questions that prompt children to think deeply and explore different possibilities helps them develop their creative problem-solving skills. For instance, asking a child, "What else could you add to this picture?" or "How do you think the story would change if the character did something different?" encourages them to consider multiple perspectives and think outside the box. These types of questions stimulate curiosity and imagination, allowing children to explore their ideas in greater depth.

Providing children with a variety of materials and experiences that inspire creativity is essential for encouraging imaginative expression. Access to a range of art supplies, building materials, books, and musical instruments gives children the tools they need to experiment with different forms of creativity. For example, offering children a choice of paints, markers, clay, or collage materials allows them to explore different artistic mediums and discover new ways to express themselves. Similarly, providing access to musical instruments or allowing children to create their own instruments from household items encourages them to experiment with sound and rhythm, fostering both creativity and cognitive development.

Hands-on activities are particularly effective in sparking creativity because they engage multiple senses and allow children to explore ideas in a tangible way. These activities provide opportunities for experimentation, problem-solving, and abstract thinking, all of which are essential for cognitive growth.

One hands-on activity that fosters creativity is building with blocks or other construction materials. Whether using wooden blocks, LEGO bricks, or natural materials like stones and sticks, children engage in creative thinking as they design and construct structures. This type of play encourages spatial reasoning, problem-solving, and engineering skills. Children must think critically about how to balance the blocks, plan their designs, and make adjustments when their structures don't work as expected. These experiences promote cognitive flexibility as children learn to adapt their plans and think creatively to solve problems.

Art projects that involve multiple steps or techniques also promote creativity and cognitive growth. For example, creating a mixed-media collage requires children to think about how to combine different textures, colors, and materials to create a cohesive artwork. This type of activity encourages children to experiment with different techniques, make decisions about composition, and use their imagination to bring their vision to life. The process of layering materials and making adjustments as they go helps children develop critical thinking skills and enhances their ability to plan and execute complex tasks.

Another hands-on activity that sparks creativity is storytelling. Encouraging children to create their own stories, either orally or in writing, helps them develop narrative skills, imagination, and critical thinking. Storytelling allows children to explore different characters, settings, and plot lines, which promotes abstract thinking and creativity. For younger children, adults can help facilitate storytelling by providing prompts or asking open-ended questions that guide the child's imagination. For older children, creative writing exercises that challenge them to think about different genres or styles of writing can help further develop their creative thinking and narrative skills.

Nature-based activities are another excellent way to foster creativity in children. Outdoor exploration allows children to engage with the natural world in imaginative and creative ways. For example, children might use natural materials like leaves, sticks, and rocks to create sculptures or mandalas, encouraging them to think creatively about how to arrange and use the materials. Nature-based art projects, such as leaf rubbings or flower pressing, allow children to explore texture, shape, and color in ways that enhance their artistic creativity. These activities also promote curiosity and inquiry, as children often ask questions about the natural world and seek to understand how things work.

Supporting artistic, musical, and dramatic play is essential for fostering creativity and cognitive benefits. These forms of creative expression allow children to explore their emotions, develop their imagination, and engage in complex problem-solving.

Artistic expression, whether through drawing, painting, sculpting, or crafting, provides children with a powerful outlet for their creativity and emotions. When children engage in artistic activities, they are not only developing their fine motor skills but also using their imagination to create something new. Art allows children to explore different ideas, experiment with color and form, and express their thoughts and feelings in a non-verbal way. This type of creative play enhances cognitive growth by encouraging children to think abstractly, make decisions about composition, and solve problems related to the artistic process.

Musical play is another important avenue for creativity and cognitive development. Music stimulates multiple areas of the brain, including those responsible for memory, attention, and language processing. Engaging in musical activities, such as playing an instrument, singing, or dancing, helps children develop rhythm, coordination, and auditory discrimination. Music also promotes creativity by encouraging children to experiment with sound, create their own melodies, and explore different musical genres. For young children, simple activities like clapping along to a beat or using household items as percussion instruments can introduce them to the concept of rhythm and sound, fostering both cognitive and creative growth.

Dramatic play, or pretend play, is one of the most powerful tools for fostering creativity and cognitive development. Through role-playing and storytelling, children create imaginary worlds where they can explore different characters, scenarios, and outcomes. This type of play encourages children to think creatively, solve problems, and understand different perspectives. For example, when children pretend to be doctors, chefs, or astronauts, they are not only using their imagination but also practicing critical thinking as they navigate the roles and responsibilities of their characters. Dramatic play also promotes social-emotional development by allowing children to explore different emotions and practice empathy as they take on different roles.

Encouraging dramatic play can be as simple as providing props and costumes that inspire imaginative scenarios. A collection of dress-up clothes, play kitchens, or toy tools can spark hours of creative play as children invent stories and take on different roles. Parents and educators can also support dramatic play by participating in the child's imaginative world, asking questions, and introducing new elements that challenge the child to think creatively and problem-solve within the context of their play.

Creative play also provides opportunities for collaborative problem-solving. When children engage in group dramatic play or collaborative art projects, they must work together to develop a shared vision, solve problems, and adapt to each other's ideas. These experiences promote cognitive flexibility and social skills, as children learn to negotiate roles, share materials, and communicate their ideas effectively. Collaborative creative play not only enhances cognitive development but also fosters important social-emotional skills, such as cooperation, empathy, and communication.

In conclusion, fostering creativity and imagination in children is essential for their cognitive, emotional, and social development. Creativity is closely linked to cognitive growth, as it encourages children to think abstractly, solve problems, and explore new ideas. By creating an environment that values creativity, offering opportunities for hands-on exploration, and supporting artistic, musical, and dramatic play, parents and educators can nurture children's creativity and help them develop the cognitive skills they need to succeed in life. Through creative expression, children develop not only their imagination but also critical thinking, problem-solving, and adaptability—skills that are essential for navigating the complexities of the modern world.

Creative activities, whether artistic, musical, or dramatic, provide an outlet for children to explore and experiment in ways that structured learning often does not allow. This freedom to innovate and think outside the box is what fosters true cognitive flexibility. As children engage in these imaginative pursuits, they are constantly challenged to assess their environment, re-imagine possibilities, and revise their approaches—key aspects of developing adaptive thinking and creativity.

In addition to cognitive benefits, creative activities provide children with important emotional outlets. By expressing their thoughts and feelings through art, music, or role-play, children are better able to process emotions and manage their internal world. Creativity gives them a way to explore complex emotions that they might not yet fully understand or have the words to express. For instance, a child who is feeling frustrated may channel those emotions into a drawing or a make-believe scenario where they have control over the narrative, helping them process their feelings in a healthy, constructive way.

Furthermore, engaging in creative activities helps children develop perseverance and resilience. Whether they are working on a painting, learning a new instrument, or trying to perfect a dance routine, creative tasks often require sustained focus and effort over time. Children learn that creativity is a process—one that sometimes involves trial and error, experimentation, and revisiting earlier steps. This experience of working through challenges builds cognitive and emotional resilience, teaching children that persistence is often the key to achieving their goals, both in creative endeavors and in life.

One of the key ways to encourage sustained creative engagement is to allow children ample time for unstructured, open-ended play. Structured activities have their place in a child's development, but it is during unstructured playtime that children are free to fully explore their creativity without the constraints of specific goals or guidelines. When children are given time and space to invent their own games, stories, and creative projects, they naturally develop problem-solving skills and learn to think flexibly.

It is also important to remember that creativity is not limited to traditional forms of artistic expression. Everyday problem-solving, such as figuring out how to build a fort with pillows and blankets or inventing new rules for a made-up game, is just as much a form of creativity as painting a picture or writing a story. Parents and educators can foster this type of creativity by encouraging children to think critically about how to approach everyday challenges in innovative ways. Instead of providing ready-made solutions, adults can ask questions like, "How do you think we could make this work?" or "What could you try next?" These questions prompt children to come up with their own ideas and solutions, fostering independent thinking and creative problem-solving.

Incorporating diverse forms of creative expression into a child's daily life also helps broaden their understanding of the world and themselves. Exposure to different forms of creativity—whether it's visual art, music, dance, drama, or even scientific inquiry—allows children to discover their unique interests and strengths. Some children may be drawn to painting and drawing, while others might find their creative outlet in writing stories, acting out plays, or experimenting with musical instruments. Providing access to a variety of creative experiences ensures that children can explore different mediums and discover what resonates with them.

Moreover, encouraging interdisciplinary creativity—where different forms of creative expression are combined—can further enhance cognitive development. For example, a child who is interested in both art and storytelling might create a picture book, combining visual and narrative elements to tell a story. Another child who enjoys music and science might experiment with creating different sounds using homemade instruments, blending their creative and analytical skills. These interdisciplinary approaches encourage children to see connections between different areas of knowledge and apply their creativity across a range of contexts.

Parents and educators play a vital role in supporting children's creative development by providing encouragement, resources, and opportunities for exploration. They can create environments that inspire curiosity and imagination, where children feel comfortable taking risks and trying new things. Importantly, fostering creativity also involves stepping back and allowing children the freedom to direct their own creative processes. Adults can offer guidance and support, but it's essential to give children the autonomy to explore their ideas and express themselves in their own unique ways.

In today's fast-paced, technology-driven world, fostering creativity is more important than ever. Creative thinking is not only a valuable skill in fields like the arts and design but is also increasingly recognized as essential for success in a wide range of professions, from engineering to entrepreneurship. Children who develop strong creative and problem-solving skills will be better equipped to navigate an ever-changing world, where adaptability, innovation, and the ability to approach challenges from multiple perspectives are crucial.

Beyond the cognitive and academic benefits, fostering creativity enriches a child's inner life and provides a lifelong source of joy and fulfillment. Whether through art, music, storytelling, or play, creativity allows children to explore their imagination, express their individuality, and make sense of the world around them. By nurturing creativity in early childhood, parents and educators not only support cognitive growth but also cultivate the creative thinkers, innovators, and problem-solvers of the future.

In summary, creativity and imagination are deeply interconnected with cognitive development, providing children with the tools they need to think critically, solve problems, and navigate the world in innovative ways. By encouraging creative thinking and expression through hands-on activities, artistic exploration, musical play, and dramatic storytelling, adults can help children develop essential cognitive skills while also fostering emotional resilience, social understanding, and a lifelong love of learning. Creativity is not only about producing art or music—it is about developing a flexible, adaptable mind capable of approaching the world with curiosity, innovation, and a sense of possibility.

Addressing Developmental Delays and Learning Disabilities

Early childhood cognitive development is a critical period that lays the foundation for lifelong learning and social functioning. While many children develop cognitive skills at a typical pace, some may experience developmental delays or learning disabilities that can affect their progress. Recognizing these challenges early on, understanding their underlying causes, and implementing effective support strategies are essential for helping children reach their full potential. This chapter will explore the importance of identifying developmental delays, the various cognitive disorders that can impact early childhood development, the role of early intervention, and the collaboration needed between parents, educators, and specialists to provide the necessary support for children facing these challenges.

Recognizing signs of developmental delays in early childhood is the first step in addressing potential learning disabilities or cognitive disorders. Developmental delays refer to when a child does not achieve developmental milestones at the expected times, which can occur in areas such as language, motor skills, social-emotional development, and cognitive functioning. These delays can vary widely in severity and may be temporary or indicative of a more persistent condition. While some children may catch up with their peers through natural development or targeted interventions, others may require ongoing support to address underlying learning disabilities.

One of the challenges in recognizing developmental delays is that early childhood development is highly individual. Children develop at different rates, and what may appear to be a delay in one child could simply be part of their unique developmental trajectory. However, there are certain signs that may indicate a more significant concern. For example, if a toddler is not using words to communicate by age two, struggles to engage with toys or objects in age-appropriate ways, or has difficulty following simple instructions, these could be signs of cognitive or language delays. Similarly, children who have trouble interacting with others, exhibit repetitive behaviors, or seem unusually detached from their surroundings may show signs of a social or emotional delay.

Parents and caregivers are often the first to notice when something does not seem quite right with a child's development. They may observe behaviors such as delayed speech, difficulty focusing on tasks, or a lack of interest in social interactions. While these behaviors can sometimes be explained by individual differences in development, they may also be indicative of an underlying cognitive disorder. It is important for parents to trust their instincts and seek professional evaluation if they are concerned about their child's progress. Early detection and intervention are crucial for addressing developmental delays and providing the support needed to help children succeed.

Cognitive disorders, such as autism spectrum disorder (ASD), attention deficit hyperactivity disorder (ADHD), and dyslexia, can significantly impact a child's cognitive development. Each of these disorders affects different aspects of cognition, learning, and behavior, and early identification is essential for implementing effective interventions.

Autism spectrum disorder (ASD) is a developmental disorder that affects social communication, behavior, and cognitive functioning. Children with autism may have difficulty with social interactions, such as making eye contact, understanding non-verbal cues, or engaging in reciprocal conversations. They may also engage in repetitive behaviors, have restricted interests, or experience sensory sensitivities. While autism affects individuals differently, with symptoms ranging from mild to severe, early signs often appear in the first few years of life. Children with autism may exhibit delays in language development, struggle with imaginative play, or show limited interest in interacting with peers. Cognitive challenges associated with autism can vary, but many children on the spectrum benefit from early intervention programs that focus on improving communication, social skills, and adaptive behaviors.

Attention deficit hyperactivity disorder (ADHD) is another cognitive disorder that can affect early childhood development. ADHD is characterized by difficulties with attention, impulsivity, and hyperactivity. Children with ADHD may have trouble staying focused on tasks, following directions, or sitting still in classroom settings. They may also struggle with self-regulation and exhibit impulsive behaviors, such as interrupting conversations or acting without thinking through the consequences. ADHD can impact a child's ability to learn and succeed in school, particularly in environments that require sustained attention and focus. Early identification and support for children with ADHD can help them develop strategies for managing their symptoms and succeeding academically.

Dyslexia is a specific learning disability that affects reading and language processing. Children with dyslexia often have difficulty decoding words, recognizing letters, and understanding the relationship between sounds and written language. As a result, they may struggle with reading fluency, comprehension, and spelling. Dyslexia is not related to intelligence, and many children with dyslexia are highly intelligent and capable learners. However, without targeted interventions, dyslexia can lead to frustration, low self-esteem, and academic difficulties. Early identification of dyslexia and the implementation of specialized reading programs can help children develop the skills they need to overcome their challenges and become confident readers.

Other cognitive disorders, such as developmental coordination disorder (DCD) or intellectual disabilities, can also impact early childhood development. DCD affects a child's ability to coordinate physical movements, making tasks like writing, dressing, or participating in sports more challenging. Intellectual disabilities involve limitations in both intellectual functioning and adaptive behaviors, affecting a child's ability to learn, reason, and function independently. Children with intellectual disabilities may require specialized educational programs that focus on developing life skills and promoting independence.

For children with developmental delays or cognitive disorders, early intervention is critical. Early intervention refers to a range of services and supports provided to children from birth to age five who have developmental delays or disabilities. These services are designed to promote development and address the specific challenges a child is facing. Early intervention can take many forms, including speech therapy, occupational therapy, physical therapy, and behavioral interventions. The goal is to provide targeted support that helps children reach developmental milestones, improve their cognitive functioning, and enhance their social-emotional development.

Research has consistently shown that early intervention is highly effective in improving outcomes for children with developmental delays and learning disabilities. The earlier a child receives intervention, the more likely they are to make significant progress in areas such as language, motor skills, and cognitive development. For example, children with autism who receive early behavioral interventions often show improvements in communication, social skills, and adaptive behaviors. Similarly, children with speech delays who participate in speech therapy can develop the language skills they need to succeed in school and everyday life.

Early intervention is also important because it helps children build the foundation for lifelong learning. Cognitive skills developed during early childhood serve as the building blocks for future academic success. By addressing developmental delays early, children are better equipped to enter school with the skills they need to thrive in the classroom. In addition, early intervention can reduce the risk of secondary problems, such as behavioral issues, low self-esteem, or difficulties with peer relationships, which can arise when developmental delays go unaddressed.

Collaboration with specialists and therapists is a key component of early intervention. Specialists, such as speech therapists, occupational therapists, physical therapists, and developmental psychologists, have expertise in addressing specific developmental challenges. They work closely with children and their families to develop individualized intervention plans that target the child's unique needs. For example, a speech therapist may work with a child to develop language skills through exercises that promote sound production, vocabulary development, and sentence structure. An occupational therapist may help a child improve fine motor skills through activities that enhance hand-eye coordination and dexterity.

Parents play an integral role in the intervention process, and collaboration between parents and specialists is essential for success. Parents are often the first to notice developmental concerns, and their observations and insights are invaluable in creating an effective intervention plan. Specialists work closely with parents to provide guidance on how to support their child's development at home, offering strategies for reinforcing the skills being taught in therapy. For example, a therapist may provide parents with exercises or activities to practice with their child between sessions, helping to reinforce progress and encourage further development.

In addition to therapists, educators play a critical role in supporting children with developmental delays and learning disabilities. Early childhood educators can collaborate with specialists to implement strategies that support a child's learning in the classroom. For example, a teacher may incorporate visual aids, hands-on activities, or alternative communication methods to help a child with autism participate in classroom activities. Educators can also provide accommodations, such as extended time for tasks or modified assignments, to ensure that children with ADHD or dyslexia can succeed academically.

For children with more significant developmental delays or disabilities, an individualized education plan (IEP) may be created to outline specific goals and services that will support the child's educational progress. IEPs are developed through collaboration between parents, educators, and specialists and are designed to meet the child's unique needs. The plan includes specific goals for the child's academic, social, and cognitive development, as well as the services and supports needed to achieve those goals. Regular meetings are held to review the child's progress and make adjustments to the plan as needed.

In addition to professional support, peer interaction is an important component of cognitive and social development for children with developmental delays. Inclusive educational environments, where children with and without disabilities learn together, provide opportunities for children to develop social skills, learn from their peers, and feel a sense of belonging. Children with developmental delays benefit from interacting with typically developing peers, while typically developing children learn empathy, patience, and an appreciation for diversity. Inclusive settings promote positive social interactions and help children with developmental delays build relationships and develop a stronger sense of self-confidence.

For families navigating developmental delays or learning disabilities, accessing support can be overwhelming. However, many resources are available to help families connect with specialists, therapies, and educational services. Early intervention programs, local education agencies, and community-based organizations often provide assessments, therapies, and resources at little to no cost. Parents are encouraged to seek support as early as possible if they have concerns about their child's development, as early action can make a significant difference in a child's cognitive and social outcomes.

In conclusion, addressing developmental delays and learning disabilities in early childhood requires a comprehensive approach that includes early recognition, targeted interventions, and collaboration between parents, specialists, and educators. By identifying developmental challenges early and providing the necessary support, children can make significant progress in their cognitive, social, and emotional development. Through early intervention, children with cognitive disorders such as autism, ADHD, and dyslexia can receive the tools they need to thrive and develop the skills necessary for lifelong success. The process of addressing developmental delays is not just about mitigating challenges but also about empowering children to reach their full potential, building on their strengths, and fostering their unique abilities. Early intervention and collaborative support help children overcome obstacles, improve their cognitive and social functioning, and prepare them for the future.

One of the most important aspects of addressing developmental delays and learning disabilities is the individualized approach that recognizes each child's unique profile of strengths and challenges. Every child's cognitive development follows its own path, and interventions must be tailored to meet the specific needs of the child. For example, a child with ADHD may benefit from behavioral strategies that help them manage their impulsivity and focus, while a child with autism may need support with social communication and sensory integration. These individualized interventions are often most effective when they are flexible and evolve with the child's progress, as developmental needs can change over time.

In addition to targeted therapies, creating a supportive home and school environment is critical for children with developmental delays or learning disabilities. Parents can create routines that help provide structure and predictability, which is especially important for children who struggle with attention, organization, or transitions between activities. Visual schedules, timers, and task charts can be helpful tools for keeping children on track and helping them understand what to expect throughout the day. Consistency in daily routines can reduce anxiety and increase a child's sense of control over their environment, making it easier for them to focus on learning and development.

In the school environment, educators play a key role in fostering a positive and inclusive atmosphere that supports children with developmental delays. Teachers who are trained to recognize the signs of developmental challenges and learning disabilities can adapt their teaching methods to accommodate the diverse needs of their students. For example, using multi-sensory teaching approaches can help children with dyslexia process information more effectively. Providing opportunities for hands-on learning, visual aids, and auditory support can cater to different learning styles and make lessons more accessible to all students.

Social-emotional development is another critical area that can be impacted by developmental delays and learning disabilities. Children who struggle with communication, attention, or social skills may find it difficult to form friendships or participate in group activities, which can lead to feelings of isolation or frustration. Supporting social-emotional development is just as important as addressing cognitive challenges, as social skills are essential for building relationships, navigating social situations, and developing a strong sense of self.

Interventions that target social-emotional development often focus on teaching children how to recognize and manage their emotions, understand social cues, and develop appropriate responses in social settings. Social skills groups, peer modeling, and play-based interventions are common approaches used to help children improve their social interactions and build meaningful connections with others. For example, role-playing scenarios or guided play can help children with autism learn how to initiate conversations, share with peers, or resolve conflicts in a positive way.

Another critical component of supporting children with developmental delays is empowering parents with knowledge and resources. Parents are a child's first and most consistent advocate, and their involvement in the intervention process is vital to the child's success. Parenting a child with developmental delays or learning disabilities can be challenging, and many parents may feel overwhelmed by the complex medical, educational, and therapeutic systems they must navigate. Providing parents with access to support networks, educational workshops, and information about available services can help them feel more confident and equipped to advocate for their child.

Collaboration between parents and professionals—whether therapists, teachers, or medical providers—is essential for creating a cohesive and comprehensive plan for the child's development. Open communication ensures that everyone involved in the child's care is working toward the same goals and using consistent strategies across different environments. Regular check-ins, progress updates, and collaborative problem-solving help keep the intervention plan on track and ensure that the child's needs are being met in a holistic way.

It is important to recognize that while children with developmental delays or learning disabilities may face additional challenges, they also have incredible potential. Many children with cognitive disorders excel in areas such as creativity, problem-solving, or specific academic subjects once they receive the right support. The goal of intervention is not just to address deficits but to unlock a child's unique strengths and help them build the skills they need to succeed in school, relationships, and life.

Inclusion is a key principle in supporting children with developmental delays or learning disabilities. An inclusive environment, whether at home, school, or in the community, ensures that all children have the opportunity to participate fully in everyday activities alongside their peers. Inclusive education, for example, allows children with disabilities to learn in the same classrooms as typically developing children, promoting social integration and reducing stigma. Inclusive practices also benefit typically developing children by fostering a sense of empathy, understanding, and respect for differences.

The success of inclusion depends on the availability of appropriate supports and accommodations. Children with developmental delays or learning disabilities may require modifications to the curriculum, additional one-on-one instruction, or the use of assistive technology to help them participate fully in classroom activities. By providing these supports, educators can create an environment where all children have the opportunity to learn, grow, and reach their potential.

Finally, it is essential to emphasize that developmental delays and learning disabilities are not indicative of a child's overall potential or ability to succeed. With early intervention, the right supports, and a collaborative approach, many children with developmental delays can make remarkable progress and achieve significant milestones. Addressing these challenges early allows children to build a strong foundation for future learning and development, empowering them to lead fulfilling and successful lives.

In conclusion, addressing developmental delays and learning disabilities in early childhood is a multifaceted process that requires early detection, targeted intervention, and collaboration between families, educators, and specialists. Recognizing the signs of developmental challenges and seeking professional evaluation is the first step in providing the support children need to thrive. By implementing individualized strategies, creating supportive environments, and fostering inclusion, we can help children overcome obstacles, build on their strengths, and develop the cognitive, social, and emotional skills they need for lifelong success.

Overcoming Socioeconomic Barriers to Cognitive Development

Socioeconomic barriers present significant challenges to early childhood cognitive development, affecting how children learn, grow, and build the foundation for future success. Poverty, in particular, has profound impacts on a child's brain development, emotional well-being, and academic potential. The limitations imposed by poverty, including limited access to educational resources, healthcare, nutritious food, and stable housing, create an environment where cognitive development can be hindered. However, with the right strategies, resources, and support, it is possible to mitigate some of the adverse effects of poverty and help children from low-income households develop the cognitive skills they need to succeed. This chapter will explore how poverty affects brain growth and learning, discuss strategies for supporting cognitive development in low-income households, and highlight resources and programs available to assist parents and educators. Additionally, it will address the importance of equity in early childhood education and how bridging the gap between socioeconomic disparities is critical for ensuring that all children, regardless of background, have equal opportunities for cognitive growth.

Poverty affects cognitive development through multiple channels, both directly and indirectly. One of the most immediate ways in which poverty impacts brain growth is through chronic stress. Children growing up in poverty are more likely to experience high levels of stress due to factors such as food insecurity, unstable housing, neighborhood violence, and parental stress. Chronic stress activates the body's stress-response system, releasing hormones such as cortisol, which, in large and prolonged amounts, can negatively affect brain development. When a child's stress response is frequently triggered, it disrupts neural connections in areas of the brain responsible for memory, attention, and emotional regulation, such as the prefrontal cortex and hippocampus. This makes it more challenging for children to focus in school, retain information, and manage their emotions, which can hinder their cognitive development and academic success.

In addition to chronic stress, poverty also limits access to the resources that are critical for healthy brain development, such as proper nutrition and healthcare. Nutrition plays a vital role in cognitive development, particularly during the early years when the brain is rapidly growing. Children in low-income households may face food insecurity or lack access to healthy, nutrient-rich foods, which can lead to deficiencies in essential nutrients like iron, omega-3 fatty acids, and vitamins that are crucial for brain development. Malnutrition, even at mild levels, can impair cognitive functions such as memory, attention, and learning capacity. Additionally, inadequate access to healthcare means that children may not receive timely medical treatment for developmental delays, hearing or vision problems, or other health issues that can affect learning and cognitive abilities.

Another significant factor is the disparity in access to early childhood education and stimulating learning environments. Children from low-income households are less likely to have access to high-quality preschools, learning materials, and extracurricular activities that foster cognitive growth. Environments rich in language, books, puzzles, and other educational toys promote cognitive development by encouraging exploration, problem-solving, and language skills. However, families living in poverty often lack the financial means to provide these enriching experiences. The so-called "word gap" phenomenon, where children from low-income families hear fewer words and have less exposure to language compared to their more affluent peers, is an example of how early exposure to language can influence cognitive development and school readiness. By the time children enter kindergarten, those from low-income backgrounds may already be at a disadvantage in terms of vocabulary, literacy, and numeracy, which affects their long-term academic performance.

While the challenges associated with poverty are significant, there are strategies that parents, educators, and communities can use to support cognitive development in low-income households. One of the most important strategies is creating a nurturing and stable environment for children, even in the face of socioeconomic hardships. Research has shown that strong, supportive relationships with caregivers can buffer the effects of chronic stress and help children develop resilience. When children feel safe and supported by their parents, they are better able to cope with the challenges they face and focus on learning. For parents in low-income households, this may mean making a conscious effort to spend quality time with their children, engaging in activities that promote bonding, such as reading together, playing, or having conversations about their day.

Incorporating routines and structure into daily life is another way to support cognitive development. Predictable routines help children feel secure and provide a framework for learning and exploration. For example, establishing a regular bedtime routine that includes reading or storytelling can promote language development and help children build the cognitive skills necessary for literacy. Similarly, setting aside time each day for play, exploration, and learning activities—whether it's drawing, building with blocks, or playing simple educational games—can stimulate cognitive growth even in resource-limited environments.

Exposure to language is one of the most critical aspects of early cognitive development, and it can be nurtured even in households with limited resources. Parents and caregivers can support language development by talking to their children regularly, reading books together, and encouraging them to express their thoughts and ideas. Simple conversations about everyday activities, like describing what they see during a walk or asking open-ended questions about their favorite toys, can enhance vocabulary and cognitive skills. If books and educational materials are not readily available, parents can make use of free community resources such as libraries, which often offer children's programs, story-time sessions, and access to a wide range of reading materials.

Access to affordable early childhood education programs is another crucial factor in supporting cognitive development for children from low-income households. Programs such as Head Start, a federal program in the United States, provide free early childhood education, health services, and nutritional support to children from disadvantaged backgrounds. These programs not only offer a stimulating learning environment but also provide children with access to essential services, such as health screenings, mental health support, and nutritional meals, which contribute to their overall cognitive and physical well-being.

Head Start and similar programs are designed to help bridge the gap between children from low-income households and their more affluent peers by providing high-quality early education that fosters cognitive development, social skills, and school readiness. Research has shown that children who participate in these programs often enter kindergarten with better language, literacy, and numeracy skills, giving them a stronger foundation for academic success.

In addition to early childhood education programs, community resources and support networks can play a significant role in helping low-income families overcome socioeconomic barriers to cognitive development. Nonprofit organizations, faith-based groups, and community centers often provide parenting workshops, educational resources, and after-school programs that offer additional learning opportunities for children. These programs may include tutoring, homework assistance, or enrichment activities such as music, art, and science projects that stimulate cognitive development. For parents who may feel isolated or overwhelmed by the challenges of poverty, these community resources can also provide valuable social support and access to services that help improve the overall well-being of the family.

Partnerships between schools, communities, and local businesses can also be instrumental in creating programs and initiatives aimed at closing the achievement gap for children from low-income households. For example, some communities have established "book banks" where families can borrow or exchange children's books for free, ensuring that even families with limited financial resources have access to reading materials. Other initiatives include free or low-cost after-school programs that provide safe, structured environments for learning and play, as well as meals for children who may not have consistent access to nutritious food at home.

Educators play a critical role in addressing the cognitive development needs of children from low-income households. Teachers in early childhood settings can implement strategies that support cognitive growth, such as differentiated instruction that meets each child's developmental level, incorporating hands-on learning experiences that engage multiple senses, and providing positive reinforcement to build self-confidence and a growth mindset. Additionally, teachers can work closely with parents to foster a collaborative approach to learning, offering guidance on how to support cognitive development at home and referring families to resources or programs that provide additional support.

Bridging the gap between socioeconomic disparities in early childhood education requires a commitment to equity. Equity in education means ensuring that all children, regardless of their socioeconomic background, have access to high-quality early learning experiences and the resources they need to thrive. It goes beyond simply providing equal opportunities and involves addressing the unique challenges faced by children from disadvantaged backgrounds, such as poverty, language barriers, or disabilities.

One of the most effective ways to promote equity in early childhood education is through targeted interventions that address the specific needs of low-income children. These interventions may include providing additional support for language development, offering free or subsidized preschool programs, and ensuring that children have access to health and nutrition services that are critical for cognitive development. Schools and educators must be equipped with the resources and training to identify and support children who are at risk of falling behind due to socioeconomic factors.

Policymakers also have a vital role to play in promoting equity in early childhood education. By investing in programs that provide comprehensive support for children from low-income households—such as universal pre-kindergarten, expanded access to Head Start, and increased funding for schools in disadvantaged areas—policymakers can help create a more level playing field for all children. Additionally, policies that address broader socioeconomic issues, such as affordable housing, healthcare access, and food security, can have a direct impact on cognitive development by reducing the stress and instability that often accompany poverty.

Addressing socioeconomic barriers to cognitive development is not just a matter of improving educational outcomes for individual children; it is also an investment in the future of society as a whole. Children who receive the support they need during their early years are more likely to succeed in school, pursue higher education, and contribute positively to their communities. Conversely, failing to address these barriers can lead to a cycle of poverty, underachievement, and limited opportunities that perpetuates inequality.

In conclusion, overcoming socioeconomic barriers to cognitive development requires a multi-faceted approach that includes supporting families, providing access to quality early childhood education, and promoting equity in education. By recognizing the impact of poverty on brain growth and learning, implementing strategies to support cognitive development in low-income households, and leveraging resources and programs available to aid parents and educators, we can help bridge the gap and ensure that all children, regardless of their socioeconomic background, have the opportunity to reach their full potential. Equity in early childhood education is essential for building a more just and equitable society, where all children, regardless of their economic circumstances, have the opportunity to succeed and thrive. By fostering environments that nurture cognitive development, offering resources that support learning, and addressing the unique challenges faced by children in poverty, we can create a foundation for lifelong success.

One of the most critical aspects of promoting equity in early childhood education is addressing the systemic barriers that disproportionately affect children from low-income households. These barriers often include inadequate funding for schools in disadvantaged areas, limited access to affordable and high-quality childcare, and a lack of trained educators who can effectively support children with diverse needs. To overcome these challenges, there must be a concerted effort to allocate resources more equitably, ensuring that children from low-income families receive the same level of educational opportunities as their more affluent peers.

At the policy level, governments can implement measures to ensure that all children have access to early learning programs, regardless of their family's financial situation. For example, expanding universal pre-kindergarten programs can help close the early achievement gap by providing every child with access to high-quality early education. Additionally, increasing funding for Head Start and similar initiatives can help low-income families access not only educational services but also health, nutrition, and family support services that are essential for cognitive development. These programs are crucial for leveling the playing field, as they provide comprehensive support that addresses the multiple factors contributing to the cognitive and academic disparities faced by children in poverty.

Another key policy area is the development of affordable, high-quality childcare options. Many low-income families struggle to find or afford reliable childcare, which can negatively impact a child's early learning experiences. When parents are forced to place their children in low-quality care settings or rely on informal childcare arrangements, children may miss out on crucial opportunities for early cognitive and social development. Investing in affordable, high-quality childcare programs can significantly improve cognitive outcomes for children in low-income households by ensuring that they receive consistent, nurturing care in environments that promote learning and development.

In addition to public policy initiatives, there are steps that individual educators and schools can take to support cognitive development and overcome socioeconomic barriers. Teachers, for example, can be trained to identify signs of developmental delays and learning difficulties early on and implement targeted interventions that address each child's needs. Professional development opportunities that focus on culturally responsive teaching, trauma-informed care, and strategies for working with children from diverse socioeconomic backgrounds can empower educators to create more inclusive and supportive learning environments.

Moreover, schools can establish partnerships with community organizations, healthcare providers, and local businesses to expand the range of resources available to low-income families. For example, a school might partner with a local clinic to provide health screenings and immunizations, or with a nonprofit organization to offer free books and learning materials to children from disadvantaged backgrounds. By building these community networks, schools can help ensure that children have access to the resources they need to thrive, both inside and outside the classroom.

Technology also has the potential to play a trans-formative role in bridging the gap between socioeconomic barriers and cognitive development. In today's digital age, access to technology can significantly enhance learning opportunities for children, particularly those in under-resourced areas. While the "digital divide" remains a significant concern—especially for low-income families who may not have access to reliable internet or digital devices—efforts to provide free or low-cost technology to disadvantaged communities are underway in many regions. Programs that provide students with tablets, laptops, or internet access can open up new avenues for learning, enabling children to access educational apps, online resources, and virtual learning platforms that support cognitive development.

However, simply providing technology is not enough. To truly make a difference, educators and parents must also be equipped with the knowledge and skills to use technology effectively in ways that promote learning and development. Schools can offer workshops and training sessions for parents and caregivers on how to use educational apps and digital tools to support their child's cognitive growth. Additionally, teachers can integrate technology into the classroom in meaningful ways, using interactive learning platforms to reinforce key concepts, promote engagement, and provide personalized learning experiences tailored to each student's needs.

In overcoming socioeconomic barriers to cognitive development, it is essential to recognize that the challenges faced by children in poverty are interconnected and multifaceted. Poverty not only limits access to material resources, but it also affects a child's emotional and psychological well-being. The stress and instability that often accompany poverty can impact a child's ability to focus, learn, and thrive in an academic setting. Addressing these challenges requires a holistic approach that considers not just educational support but also mental health services, family support programs, and initiatives that promote stability and security for low-income families.

For example, mental health services can play a crucial role in supporting children who have experienced trauma or chronic stress due to poverty. Early intervention programs that provide counseling, social-emotional learning, and behavioral support can help children develop coping skills and emotional resilience, which are essential for cognitive development. Schools can work with mental health professionals to create trauma-informed classrooms that recognize the impact of poverty-related stress on learning and behavior, and provide strategies for helping children feel safe, supported, and ready to learn.

Family support programs are another critical component of overcoming socioeconomic barriers. Initiatives that provide parenting education, financial literacy training, and job assistance for parents can help improve family stability and create an environment that is conducive to learning and development. When parents have the resources and support they need to provide a stable home environment, children are more likely to thrive both cognitively and emotionally. Programs that offer home visits, early literacy support, and guidance on child development can empower parents to play an active role in their child's education and ensure that they are equipped with the knowledge and tools to support their child's cognitive growth.

Ultimately, overcoming the socioeconomic barriers to cognitive development requires a collective effort from parents, educators, policymakers, and communities. By addressing the root causes of poverty and investing in comprehensive support systems that prioritize early childhood education and cognitive development, we can create a more equitable society where all children have the opportunity to succeed. It is not enough to simply provide equal access to education; we must also ensure that children from disadvantaged backgrounds have the support and resources they need to overcome the unique challenges they face.

Equity in early childhood education is about more than just closing the achievement gap—it is about creating a world where every child, regardless of their socioeconomic status, has the chance to reach their full potential. Through targeted interventions, policy changes, and a commitment to providing high-quality, inclusive education for all, we can help bridge the gap and ensure that every child has the opportunity to build a strong foundation for lifelong learning and success.

Transitioning from Early Childhood to School Age

T ransitioning from early childhood to school age is a significant milestone in a child's cognitive, social, and emotional development. This transition marks the beginning of formal education and sets the stage for future learning experiences. For children, entering kindergarten or first grade can bring excitement and challenges as they adjust to new routines, expectations, and environments. The cognitive development that occurs during early childhood (from birth to age five) provides a foundation for school readiness, but cognitive growth continues beyond this period as children engage in increasingly complex thinking and problem-solving tasks. This chapter will explore the process of preparing for kindergarten and first grade, examine how cognitive development evolves beyond age five, discuss strategies for encouraging lifelong learning habits, and highlight the importance of building a growth mindset to support a child's continued success.

Preparing for kindergarten and first grade involves much more than simply learning academic skills like recognizing letters and numbers. While these early literacy and numeracy skills are important, school readiness encompasses a broad range of cognitive, social, emotional, and physical abilities that help children succeed in a structured school environment. Preparing a child for this transition involves fostering the skills and behaviors that enable them to navigate the challenges of formal education, such as the ability to follow directions, focus on tasks, solve problems, and interact positively with peers and teachers.

One of the most critical aspects of preparing for kindergarten is developing self-regulation skills. Self-regulation refers to a child's ability to manage their emotions, behavior, and attention in response to the demands of their environment. In a classroom setting, children are expected to follow rules, take turns, listen to instructions, and manage their impulses. For young children, learning how to regulate their behavior in these ways can be challenging, especially in a new and structured environment like a classroom. Parents and caregivers can support the development of self-regulation by providing opportunities for children to practice these skills at home. Simple activities such as playing board games (which require taking turns and following rules), engaging in pretend play (which encourages role-playing and perspective-taking), and participating in group activities (which promote patience and cooperation) help children build the skills they need to thrive in a classroom setting.

Another important component of school readiness is language development. Children who enter kindergarten with strong language skills are better equipped to communicate with their peers and teachers, understand instructions, and engage in learning activities. To support language development, parents and caregivers can encourage conversation, storytelling, and reading at home. Asking open-ended questions that prompt children to think and articulate their ideas, reading a variety of books together, and discussing new vocabulary are all effective ways to enhance language skills. Additionally, children benefit from being exposed to rich and varied language environments, where they have opportunities to hear and use language in meaningful ways.

Social-emotional development is also a key factor in preparing for school. Children who have strong social skills, such as the ability to share, cooperate, and resolve conflicts, are more likely to have positive experiences in kindergarten and first grade. Social-emotional learning (SEL) programs, which teach children how to manage their emotions, build positive relationships, and make responsible decisions, are becoming more common in early childhood education settings. Parents can support this aspect of development by modeling positive social interactions, helping children identify and express their emotions, and providing guidance on how to handle challenging social situations.

Additionally, building early problem-solving and critical thinking skills is essential for school readiness. In kindergarten and first grade, children are expected to engage in tasks that require higher-order thinking, such as sorting, classifying, comparing, and making predictions. These skills can be developed through play and everyday activities that challenge children to think critically about the world around them. For example, puzzles, building blocks, and games that involve strategy encourage children to use logic, reasoning, and creativity to solve problems. Providing opportunities for open-ended play, where children can explore different possibilities and experiment with solutions, fosters the development of these cognitive skills.

Physical readiness for school is also important, as fine motor skills (such as holding a pencil, cutting with scissors, or manipulating small objects) are necessary for many classroom tasks. Activities like drawing, coloring, and playing with clay or building materials can help children strengthen their fine motor skills in preparation for writing and other school-related tasks. Gross motor skills, such as running, jumping, and balancing, are also important for overall physical health and well-being and can be developed through active play and outdoor exploration.

As children transition from early childhood to school age, cognitive development continues to evolve in significant ways. While the early years lay the foundation for learning, the cognitive growth that occurs during the school years builds on these early experiences and prepares children for more complex thinking and learning in later stages of life.

One of the major changes in cognitive development beyond age five is the shift from concrete to more abstract thinking. In early childhood, children primarily rely on concrete experiences to understand the world. They learn through direct interaction with their environment, using their senses to explore and make sense of objects and events. As they move into the school years, however, children begin to develop the ability to think more abstractly. They can understand and manipulate concepts that are not directly tied to physical objects, such as numbers, letters, and symbols. This shift is essential for learning academic subjects like mathematics, reading, and science, where abstract thinking plays a key role.

Memory also plays a crucial role in cognitive development during the school years. Children develop better working memory, which allows them to hold and manipulate information in their minds over short periods of time. This ability is important for tasks such as following multi-step instructions, solving math problems, and reading comprehension. Additionally, long-term memory improves, allowing children to retain information over extended periods and apply what they have learned to new situations. Encouraging children to practice memory-building activities, such as recalling details from a story or remembering sequences of events, can support the development of both working and long-term memory.

Another key aspect of cognitive development beyond age five is the continued growth of executive function skills. Executive functions, which include planning, organizing, prioritizing, and self-monitoring, are critical for academic success and everyday life. These skills help children set goals, manage their time, and adapt to changing circumstances. For example, when a child is faced with a difficult homework assignment, strong executive function skills allow them to break the task into smaller steps, organize their materials, and monitor their progress. Parents and educators can support the development of executive functions by providing opportunities for children to practice these skills in real-life contexts, such as organizing a project, planning a schedule, or reflecting on their performance after completing a task.

Encouraging lifelong learning habits is one of the most important goals during the transition from early childhood to school age. Lifelong learning is the idea that learning is a continuous process that extends beyond formal education and into all aspects of life. Children who develop a love of learning and curiosity about the world are more likely to seek out new knowledge and experiences throughout their lives.

One of the most effective ways to encourage lifelong learning is by fostering a sense of curiosity and exploration. Children are naturally curious, and parents and educators can nurture this curiosity by providing opportunities for discovery and inquiry. Whether it's exploring nature, asking questions about how things work, or engaging in creative problem-solving, encouraging children to follow their interests and investigate the world around them helps them develop a mindset that values learning as an ongoing process.

Creating a positive attitude toward learning is also essential. Children who feel confident in their ability to learn and who see learning as enjoyable are more likely to embrace new challenges and persist when faced with difficulties. Praise for effort, rather than just for success, reinforces the idea that learning is a journey and that mistakes are part of the process. When children understand that they can improve through practice and persistence, they are more likely to take risks and try new things. Parents can support this by providing positive feedback that focuses on growth, such as, "I can see how hard you're working on this puzzle. You're getting better and better at figuring it out!"

Another key aspect of fostering lifelong learning is providing children with diverse learning experiences. Exposing children to different subjects, activities, and perspectives broadens their understanding of the world and encourages them to explore new areas of interest. For example, parents and educators can introduce children to various types of books, art, music, science experiments, and cultural experiences, helping them discover new passions and hobbies. Encouraging participation in extracurricular activities, such as sports, clubs, or community service, also provides opportunities for learning outside the classroom and fosters a well-rounded approach to education.

Building a growth mindset is a crucial element of supporting cognitive development and encouraging lifelong learning. A growth mindset is the belief that intelligence and abilities can be developed through effort, practice, and learning from mistakes. This mindset contrasts with a fixed mindset, where individuals believe that their intelligence and talents are static traits that cannot change.

Research has shown that children with a growth mindset are more likely to embrace challenges, persist in the face of obstacles, and view effort as a path to mastery. They are less likely to be discouraged by failure and more likely to see mistakes as opportunities to learn and grow. In contrast, children with a fixed mindset may avoid challenges, give up easily, and feel threatened by failure, believing that their abilities are fixed and cannot be improved.

Parents and educators play a key role in shaping a child's mindset by the way they provide feedback and encouragement. Praise that focuses on effort, strategy, and perseverance fosters a growth mindset, while praise that focuses solely on innate abilities (such as telling a child they are "smart") can inadvertently reinforce a fixed mindset. For example, saying, "You worked so hard to figure that out!" emphasizes the importance of effort, while saying, "You're so smart!" may lead a child to believe that their success is due to an unchangeable trait rather than their hard work.

In addition to providing growth-oriented feedback, adults can model a growth mindset by sharing their own experiences with learning and per-sistence. For instance, if a parent or teacher encounters a challenge, they can talk about how they approached the problem, made mistakes, and ultimately found a solution. This kind of modeling shows children that learning is a process that involves setbacks and persistence, which are normal parts of growth. By observing adults who approach challenges with a positive and determined mindset, children learn that their own abilities can be improved through hard work and dedication.

An important part of fostering a growth mindset is teaching children how to set realistic and achievable goals. Goal-setting helps children understand that progress comes in steps and that reaching a large goal often involves breaking it down into smaller, manageable tasks. For example, if a child is learning to read, setting smaller goals like mastering a set of sight words or reading a short book can provide a sense of accomplishment and keep them motivated. As children achieve these smaller goals, they gain confidence in their abilities and are more likely to take on larger challenges in the future.

Building resilience is another key aspect of developing a growth mindset. Resilience refers to the ability to bounce back from failure or disappointment and continue moving forward. Children who are resilient are more likely to view failure as a temporary setback rather than a reflection of their abilities. To help children build resilience, parents and educators can encourage them to reflect on their experiences, identify what went wrong, and think about how they might approach a problem differently next time. This process of reflection and adjustment fosters a sense of ownership over their learning and helps children develop problem-solving skills that will serve them throughout their lives.

Encouraging children to take risks and try new things is also important for fostering a growth mindset. When children are given the freedom to experiment, make mistakes, and learn from their experiences, they develop the confidence to tackle new challenges. Parents and educators can create a safe and supportive environment where children feel comfortable taking risks without fear of judgment or failure. For example, in a classroom setting, teachers can design activities that encourage exploration and creativity, where the focus is on the learning process rather than the final product.

Another way to build a growth mindset is through the use of language that emphasizes learning and effort over innate talent. For example, instead of praising a child for being "a natural" at a particular subject, adults can emphasize the hard work and perseverance that contributed to the child's success. This approach reinforces the idea that abilities can be developed and that success is the result of effort rather than fixed traits. Additionally, when children encounter difficulties, encouraging them to use phrases like "I can't do this yet" rather than "I can't do this" helps them understand that learning is a process and that improvement is possible with practice.

As children transition from early childhood to school age, it is important to continue supporting their cognitive development through activities that challenge their thinking and promote problem-solving. One effective strategy for doing this is to provide children with opportunities for open-ended play and exploration. Activities that allow children to experiment, make choices, and solve problems on their own promote cognitive flexibility and critical thinking. For example, building with blocks, creating art projects, or engaging in role-playing games all require children to use their imagination, think critically, and come up with creative solutions to challenges.

In addition to open-ended play, structured learning activities can also support cognitive development and foster a growth mindset. Educational games, puzzles, and activities that require children to use logic, reasoning, and planning are valuable tools for promoting cognitive growth. For example, games that involve strategy, such as chess or board games, challenge children to think ahead and make decisions based on available information. These types of activities not only build cognitive skills but also teach children how to approach problems systematically and learn from their mistakes.

Another important aspect of promoting cognitive development during the school years is providing children with opportunities to practice self-directed learning. Self-directed learning encourages children to take ownership of their education by setting their own goals, seeking out information, and reflecting on their progress. This approach fosters independence and a sense of responsibility for one's own learning. For example, parents and educators can encourage children to pursue projects or topics that interest them, whether it's researching a favorite animal, building a model, or writing a story. By allowing children to explore their passions and set their own learning goals, adults help them develop the skills and confidence needed for lifelong learning.

Fostering collaboration and peer learning is another effective way to promote cognitive development and build a growth mindset. Working with others allows children to learn from different perspectives, share ideas, and solve problems collaboratively. Group projects, discussions, and cooperative learning activities encourage children to communicate, negotiate, and think critically about how to approach challenges. In addition, peer learning provides opportunities for children to model positive behaviors, such as perseverance and resilience, for one another. When children see their peers trying hard, learning from mistakes, and celebrating successes, they are more likely to adopt these attitudes in their own learning.

As children move from early childhood to school age, the development of executive function skills becomes increasingly important. Executive functions, which include planning, organization, time management, and self-regulation, are critical for academic success and everyday life. Helping children develop these skills prepares them to handle the more complex demands of school and beyond.

Parents and educators can support the development of executive functions by providing children with opportunities to practice planning and organizing tasks. For example, parents might involve children in planning a family activity, such as organizing a trip to the zoo or preparing for a birthday party. These tasks require children to think ahead, make decisions, and prioritize steps to achieve a goal. In the classroom, teachers can incorporate activities that require students to plan, such as organizing a research project or setting up a science experiment. These types of activities help children develop the cognitive skills necessary for managing tasks and following through on goals.

Time management is another critical executive function skill that can be fostered during the transition to school age. Children who learn how to manage their time effectively are better able to balance schoolwork, extracurricular activities, and free time. Parents can help children develop time management skills by establishing routines that provide structure for homework, chores, and play. Additionally, providing children with visual tools, such as calendars or timers, can help them track their progress and manage their time more effectively.

As children continue to develop their executive functions, self-regulation becomes increasingly important. Self-regulation involves the ability to control impulses, stay focused on tasks, and manage emotions in response to challenges. Children who have strong self-regulation skills are better equipped to handle frustration, stay on task, and adapt to changing circumstances. To support self-regulation, parents and educators can provide children with strategies for managing their emotions and staying focused. For example, teaching mindfulness techniques, such as deep breathing or taking a break when feeling overwhelmed, can help children calm themselves and refocus their attention. Additionally, providing clear expectations and routines helps children understand what is expected of them and develop the self-discipline needed to stay on track.

In conclusion, the transition from early childhood to school age is a critical period of cognitive, social, and emotional growth. Preparing for kindergarten and first grade involves fostering self-regulation, language development, and problem-solving skills, while cognitive development continues to evolve beyond age five through the growth of abstract thinking, memory, and executive function skills. Encouraging lifelong learning habits, fostering a growth mindset, and providing opportunities for exploration, collaboration, and self-directed learning are essential for helping children succeed in school and beyond. By supporting children during this important transition, parents, educators, and caregivers can help lay the foundation for a lifetime of learning and growth.

Conclusion

Supporting cognitive development in children is one of the most vital responsibilities parents, caregivers, and educators undertake. It's a journey filled with daily opportunities to nurture, encourage, and guide children through various stages of growth. Throughout this book, we've explored key factors, strategies, and insights that shape a child's cognitive abilities from early childhood through the transition to school age. The overarching goal has been to empower adults with the knowledge and tools necessary to help children develop essential thinking skills, emotional resilience, and a love for learning that will serve them for life.

Reflecting on the key takeaways from this book highlights the multifaceted nature of cognitive development. It's clear that the early years are critical for brain growth, but cognitive development is not confined to the early childhood period. It continues to evolve as children mature, learn, and interact with their environments. We've covered how various factors such as nutrition, social interactions, play, language, and early learning experiences contribute to brain development and cognitive abilities. Understanding these elements is important for providing the right kind of support and stimulation to foster a child's cognitive growth.

One of the most important takeaways is the powerful role of the environment in shaping cognitive development. From the home to the classroom, children's surroundings play a crucial role in their cognitive, emotional, and social development. A nurturing and stimulating environment, where children feel safe to explore, experiment, and make mistakes, is essential for promoting brain growth and cognitive skills. In this type of environment, children are encouraged to ask questions, solve problems, and engage with the world around them. We've discussed the importance of play, language-rich interactions, and supportive relationships as key elements that nurture a child's developing brain.

Another major theme is the role of early intervention and support when cognitive challenges or developmental delays arise. Recognizing the signs of developmental delays and seeking help early can make a significant difference in a child's cognitive outcomes. Whether addressing language delays, attention difficulties, or learning disabilities, early intervention offers the tools and resources needed to provide children with the support they need to thrive. Parents, caregivers, and educators are encouraged to be proactive, seek professional advice when needed, and collaborate with specialists to ensure children receive the right kind of help.

The importance of developing executive function skills, such as self-regulation, working memory, and cognitive flexibility, has also been a central focus. These skills are essential for school readiness, academic success, and everyday problem-solving. We've explored how structured routines, goal-setting, and opportunities for decision-making can help children strengthen their executive function skills, enabling them to manage tasks, make thoughtful decisions, and adapt to new challenges.

Consistency and patience are key when it comes to supporting cognitive development. Children's growth is a gradual process, and it can sometimes be difficult to see immediate results. However, the small, everyday interactions you have with your child—whether it's reading together, engaging in play, or having meaningful conversations—are laying the groundwork for long-term cognitive development. By consistently providing opportunities for exploration, learning, and problem-solving, you are helping your child build the skills they need to succeed.

Patience is equally important, especially when children encounter challenges or difficulties in their development. It's natural for children to struggle at times, whether with learning new concepts, managing emotions, or interacting with others. As a parent or caregiver, offering patience, understanding, and support during these moments helps children build resilience and develop a positive mindset toward learning. Rather than focusing solely on outcomes, it's important to celebrate effort, perseverance, and progress. This approach not only fosters a growth mindset but also helps children develop confidence in their abilities and a willingness to take on new challenges.

Creating a future full of potential for your child requires a commitment to fostering a love of learning and a sense of curiosity about the world. One of the most effective ways to do this is by being an active participant in your child's learning journey. Show interest in their questions, engage in conversations about their experiences, and provide encouragement as they explore new ideas. Whether it's asking them about their day at school, participating in hands-on activities, or guiding them through a new project, your involvement plays a crucial role in shaping your child's attitude toward learning.

A future full of potential also means helping children develop the social-emotional skills they need to succeed in life. Cognitive development is not just about academic success—it's also about building strong relationships, managing emotions, and developing empathy. By creating an environment where children feel valued, respected, and supported, you are helping them develop the social-emotional foundation they need to thrive. Encouraging cooperative play, teaching conflict resolution skills, and modeling positive social interactions are all ways to help children build strong social-emotional skills.

As parents, caregivers, and educators, it's essential to remember that you are your child's first and most important teacher. The experiences, interactions, and opportunities you provide have a profound impact on your child's cognitive development. Your role is not only to teach academic skills but also to inspire curiosity, foster creativity, and nurture a love of learning. By being present, engaged, and supportive, you are helping your child develop the cognitive, emotional, and social skills they need to navigate life's challenges and achieve their full potential.

It's important to recognize that supporting cognitive development is a lifelong process. While the early years are critical, cognitive growth continues well beyond childhood. The skills, attitudes, and habits children develop during these formative years will serve them throughout their lives. By fostering a growth mindset, encouraging curiosity, and providing opportunities for exploration and learning, you are laying the foundation for lifelong cognitive development. This means being open to new experiences, embracing challenges, and continuing to learn and grow alongside your child.

For educators, your role extends beyond teaching academic content. You are shaping the minds of the next generation, creating an environment where children feel empowered to explore, ask questions, and take risks in their learning. Your encouragement and support can make a lasting impact on a child's cognitive development. By providing engaging, hands-on learning experiences, fostering collaboration, and offering positive reinforcement, you help children develop a love of learning that will last a lifetime.

Finally, a word of encouragement for parents, caregivers, and educators: the work you do is invaluable. Supporting a child's cognitive development is not always easy, and there will undoubtedly be challenges along the way. However, the time, effort, and dedication you invest in your child's growth and learning are some of the most important contributions you can make to their future. Every interaction, every moment of guidance, and every opportunity for exploration you provide helps shape the person your child will become.

In moments when progress seems slow or challenges arise, remember that cognitive development is a marathon, not a sprint. Be patient with yourself and your child, and trust that the consistent support you provide will yield long-term benefits. Celebrate the small victories, and keep in mind that learning is a process that involves ups and downs. By staying committed to your child's development, you are helping them build the skills, confidence, and mindset they need to succeed.

In conclusion, your role in supporting cognitive development is both powerful and profound. Through your actions, words, and guidance, you are shaping your child's brain, helping them build the cognitive skills that will enable them to succeed academically, socially, and emotionally. Whether you're a parent, caregiver, or educator, your commitment to fostering cognitive development makes a lasting impact on your child's life.

As you move forward, keep the key takeaways from this book in mind: the importance of a supportive and stimulating environment, the value of early intervention and collaboration with specialists, the power of consistency and patience, and the significance of building a growth mindset. Together, these elements create a solid foundation for cognitive growth and lifelong learning. By being present, engaged, and supportive, you are helping your child reach their full potential and creating a future full of possibilities.

Keep nurturing your child's curiosity, keep encouraging their efforts, and remember that your role in their cognitive development is one of the most important and rewarding journeys you will ever embark upon. Your love, guidance, and support are the greatest gifts you can give your child as they navigate the path of learning, growth, and discovery.